2 Manuscripts

The Art of Intermittent Fasting:
How to Lose Weight, Burn Fat, and Live a Healthier Life

&

The Ultimate Fasting Diet:
Simple Intermittent Fasting Strategies to Boost Weight Loss, Control Hunger, Fight Disease, and Slow Down Aging
(Comes with 28 Easy, Fast, and Delicious Recipes)

Table of Contents

Book 1

The Art of Intermittent Fasting: *How to Lose Weight, Shed Fat, and Live a Healthier Life*

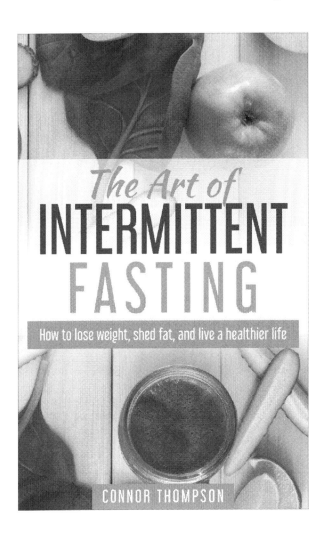

Introduction

Congratulations on downloading this book and thank you for doing so.

The following chapters will discuss everything that you need to know to get started with intermittent fasting. This is a great diet plan that focuses more on the time to eat foods as opposed to the actual food you are eating. There are also a wide variety of options when it comes to using the intermittent fast so you will be able to make it work for your lifestyle.

This guidebook will provide you with all the information that you need to get started with an intermittent fast. We will look at what this fast is all about, the health benefits that come with it, how to eat on this diet plan, and much more. We will also answer some common questions about fasting so that you are fully prepared to get started.

The intermittent fast can be a great option for those who have had trouble losing weight in the past and who want something that will actually work well for them now. Make sure to check out this guidebook to help you to get started with intermittent fasting today.

There are plenty of books on this subject on the market so thanks again for choosing this one. Every effort was made to ensure it is packed full of useful information so please enjoy!

Chapter 1: How Our Modern Diet is Failing Us

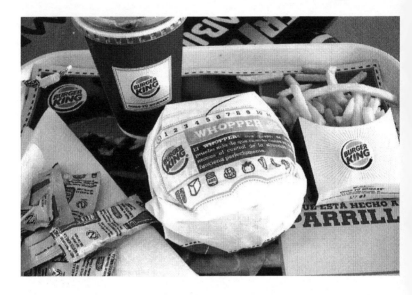

We all know that we need to eat healthier. We also know that we need to limit how much soda, juice, processed foods, sugars that we consume. But even though we know these things, it doesn't mean that it is as easy to follow.

According to a recent food and health survey done by Psychology Today, 52 percent of Americans believe that it is easier for them to figure out their taxes than to figure out how to eat healthily. Plenty of people have trouble with the current tax code, which means even more people are having trouble figuring out how to eat a diet that is good for them.

We live in a country that is fighting a battle with obesity. More than a third of the population in the United States is considered obese, and many are also considered overweight. However, these statistics do not show the complete picture. Two out of three adults are considered overweight or obese, meaning that most people will fall into this category.

Why are these statistics so dismal? There are a lot of factors that contribute to obesity. One big culprit is the standard American diet. There has been a huge decrease in the quality of our diets as we went from a nation that relied on food from local farms to a nation that mass-produces most of our food. This transition has increased our food consumption because it is so readily available now.

In addition, many foods that are readily available and easy to eat are high in fat, sugars, and calories. All of these things contribute to added weight. From the sugary snacks that we find in the break room to all the fast food chains that are around us, the quality of food and the amount we eat has changed drastically. We can literally eat unhealthy foods non-stop if we wish, which is why obesity is so prevalent in our culture.

The first thing we should look at is the quantity of food that we are eating. The number of calories that each person needs varies from person to person. Factors include your genetics, activity level, overall health, height, age, and gender. However, the benchmark number that is used on food labels is about 2000 calories each day. This number is already fairly high for those who live a sedentary life. It is also possible to eat 2000 calories or more in just one sitting if you go out to eat.

While eating out quickly pushes us past calorie limits, it is also possible to eat more even when we eat at home. It is important to learn how to start eating what we need to function, rather than eating because something tastes good, or we are bored, tired, or sad.

To calculate the average amount of daily calories that are consumed by Americans, organizations examine the amount of food available per person as indicators for the amount of food that is consumed. Inside the United States, this ends up being around 3800 calories each day. Even when you account for the fact that some of this food is wasted or discarded each day rather than consumed, the average American still consumes 2700 calories each day. This is way more than anyone will need, even if they are leading an active lifestyle, which many Americans are not.

Now, we need to also discuss the quality of the food that most Americans are eating. Growing up, most of us learn from our parents and teachers which foods are good and which ones are not. Fruits and vegetables are seen as good, and sugars and sweets are bad. The rest of the foods may not have been as good for you, but they were fine in moderation. Even though we were taught about healthy eating at a young age, in practice, it is much harder to follow this advice.

According to the U.S. Department of Agriculture, the top six sources of calories for most Americans are grain-based desserts, yeast bread, chicken, soda/sports and energy drinks, and alcoholic beverages. Note that healthy fruits and vegetables are not listed. Out of this top five list, most of the foods that Americans consume are refined grains and sugars. It is estimated that only 8% of the average American diet consists of fruits and vegetables.

According to a study done by the United States Department of Agriculture (USDA) in 2010, nuts, meats, and eggs make up 21% of these diets; oils and fats are 23%, and caloric sweeteners make up 15%. The food that is not that good for us makes up a good 61 percent of our diets.

The time of day that we eat can matter as well. Most Americans live a busy lifestyle, and they do not have the time to sit down and eat a well-balanced meal. Instead, they eat on the go, usually at some place that is unhealthy, or they eat at night when their metabolisms are slower. In addition, many Americans are sitting on the couch and eating unhealthy snack foods while watching television. Sometimes food is so abundant that we eat non-stop.

It is important to learn the necessary steps to limit how much food we are taking in each day. It is tempting to eat foods that are easily available. But, if you want to regain your health and stay in good shape, it is important to step away from the typical American diet and choose something that is healthier and better for you.

When you hear about fasting, you might think of people who go for weeks without eating due to religious reasons. You might think that it is unhealthy or that you won't be able to do it since you love food too much. But intermittent fasting is different from religious fasting, although they do share some common ideas.

Intermittent fasting is about restricting your calorie intake during certain parts of the day or not eating as much on certain days. Your body still gets the nutrients it needs, but you eat fewer calories, therefore making it is easier to lose weight. Some of the different types of intermittent fasting will be discussed later on in the book.

The reason why this diet is successful is that it is effective at reducing the amount of fat that is in your body as well as the number of calories that you are consuming. Since you are reducing the time frame in which you are allowed to eat or lowering your calorie intake during certain days of the week, it is much easier to lower the calorie count overall.

You can also choose how long you would like to do the intermittent fast. Some people choose to do it for a month or more while others fit it into their lifestyles, so they stick with it long term.

Chapter 2: What is Intermittent Fasting

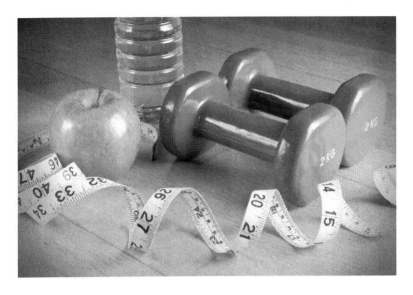

Now that we have taken some time to look at how the American diet is making us unhealthy, let's look an eating style that will make it easier to lose weight and become healthier. This chapter will discuss what intermittent fasting is all about so you can understand how it may work for you.

Intermittent fasting consists of a dieter cycling between periods when they are allowed to eat and periods where they are supposed to fast. This type of diet doesn't necessarily say which foods you can eat but specifies when you should eat. Of course, if you want to lose weight or get a better health, it is better to eat foods that are good for you and nutritious. However, with intermittent fasting, it's not going to specifically list out which foods you can and cannot have.

There are different types of intermittent fasting methods, but all of them split up your day or week into eating periods and fasting periods. What you may be surprised to know is that most of us already fast each day when we are sleeping. You could extend the natural fast time for a little bit longer. For example, you may decide to skip breakfast and have your first meal at noon and your last meal at 8 pm. This would be considered a form of intermittent fasting.

With this method, you technically fast for sixteen hours each day and then only eat during an eight-hour period of the day. This form of fasting, also known as the 16/8 method, is one of the popular options when it comes to intermittent fasting.

Despite what you may be thinking right now, intermittent fasting is actually easier than you think. It doesn't take much planning and countless people who have gone on this diet report that they feel better and have more energy when they are on a fast. In the beginning, you may struggle a bit with hunger, but it won't take long before your body adapts and gets used to it.

The main thing to remember is that when you are in the fasting period, you are not allowed to eat. You can still drink beverages to keep you hydrated. Some of the options include tea, coffee, water, and other non-caloric beverages. Some forms of this fast will allow for a bit of food during the fasting periods, but most don't. And if you like, it is usually fine to take a supplement while you are on this fast, as long as it doesn't contain calories.

Why fast?

The next question that you may have is why you should consider fasting in the first place. Humans have actually been going through periods of fasting for many years. Sometimes they did this because it was a necessity since they were not able to find any food to eat. Then there were also times that the fasting was done for religious reasons. Religions such as Buddhism, Christianity, and Islam mandate some form of fasting. Also, it is natural to fast when you are feeling sick.

Although fasting sometimes has a negative connotation, there is really nothing that is unnatural about fasting. In fact, our bodies are well equipped to handle times when we have to go without eating. There are quite a few processes inside of the body that changes when we go on a fast. This helps our bodies to continue functioning during periods of famine.

When we fast, we get a significant reduction in insulin and blood sugar levels, as well as a drastic increase in what is known as the human growth hormone. While this was something that was originally done when food was scarce, it is now used to help people to lose weight. With fasting, burning fat becomes simple, easier, and effective.

Some people decide to go on a fast because it can help their metabolism. This kind of fasting is good for improving various health disorders and diseases. There is also some evidence that shows how intermittent fasting can help you to live longer. Studies show that rodents were able to extend their lifespan with intermittent fasting.

Other research shows that fasting can help protect against various diseases such as Alzheimer's, cancer, type-2 diabetes, and heart disease. And then there are those who choose to go on an intermittent fast because it's convenient for their lifestyle. Fasting can be a really effective life hack. For instance, the fewer meals you have to make, the simpler your life will become.

Why does intermittent fasting work?

Intermittent fasting is the practice of scheduling your meals in order for your body to get the most out of them. Rather than cutting your calorie intake in half, depriving yourself of all the foods you enjoy, or diving into a trendy diet fad, intermittent fasting is a simple, logical, and healthful way of eating that promotes fat loss. There are many ways to approach intermittent fasting, but it's basically defined as a specific eating pattern. This method focuses on changing when you eat, rather than what you eat.

When you begin intermittent fasting, you will most likely keep your calorie intake the same, but rather than spreading your meals throughout the day, you will eat bigger meals during a shorter time frame. For example, rather than eating 3 to 4 meals a day, you might eat one large meal at 11 am, then another large meal at 6 pm, with no meals in between 11 am and 6 pm, and after 6 pm, no meals until 11 am the next day. This is only one method of intermittent fasting, and others will be detailed in this book in later chapters. However, you first must understand why this method works.

Intermittent fasting is a method utilized by many bodybuilders, athletes, and fitness gurus to keep their muscle mass high and their body fat percentage low. It is a simple strategy that allows you to eat the foods you enjoy, while still promoting fat loss and muscle gain or maintenance. Intermittent fasting can be practiced short term or long term, but the best results come from adopting this method into your daily lifestyle.

Though the word "fasting" may make alarm the average person, intermittent fasting does not equate to starving yourself. To understand the principals behind successful intermittent fasting, we'll first go over the body's two states digestion: the fed state and the fasting state.

For three to five hours after eating a meal, your body is in what is known as the "fed state." During the fed state, your insulin levels increase to absorb and digest your food. When your insulin levels are high, it is very difficult for your body to burn fat. Insulin is a hormone produced by the pancreas to regulate glucose levels in the bloodstream. Though its purpose is to regulate, insulin is technically a storage hormone. When insulin levels are high, your body is burning your food for energy, rather than your stored fat which is why increased levels of it prevent weight loss.

After the three to five hours are up, your body has finished processing the meal, and you enter the post-absorptive state. The post-absorptive state lasts anywhere from 8 to 12 hours. After this time gap is when your body enters the fasted state. Since your body has completely processed your food by this point, your insulin levels are low, making your stored fat extremely accessible for burning.

In the fasted state, your body has no food left to utilized for energy, so your stored fat is burned instead. Intermittent fasting allows your body to reach an advanced fat burning state that you would normally reach with the average, 'three meals per day' eating pattern. This factor alone is the reason why many people notice rapid results with intermittent fasting without even making changes to their exercise routines, how much they eat, or what they eat. They are simply changing the timing and pattern of their food intake.

When you begin an intermittent fasting program, it may take some time to get into the swing of things. Don't get discouraged! If you slip up, just get back into your intermittent fasting pattern when you can. Avoid beating yourself up, or feeling guilty. Negative self-talk will only prolong you getting back to your pattern. Making a lifestyle change takes a conscious effort, and no one expects you to do it perfectly right away. If you are not used to going long periods without eating, intermittent fasting will take some getting used to. As long as you choose the right method for you, stay focused and remain positive, you will get the hang of it in no time.

Unlike some of the other diet plans that you may go on, the intermittent fast is one that will work. It uses your body and how it works to its advantage to help you to really lose weight. It is easy to get a bit scared when you hear about fasting. You may assume that you need to spend days and weeks without eating (and who really has the willpower to give up their food for that long even when they do want to lose weight) and that it will be too hard for you.

Intermittent fasting is a bit different than you may imagine. Not only is it really hard to go on a fast for weeks at a time, but it is also not good for the body. Your body will often go into starvation mode if you end up being on the fast for too long. It assumes that you are in a time without much food and so the body will work on saving the calories and helping you to hold on to the fat and calories for as long as possible.

This means that not only are you hungry, but you are also missing out on losing weight.

You don't have to get too worried about how this intermittent fast will work in the starvation mode. The intermittent fast is effective because you are not going to fast for so long that the body goes into this starvation mode and stops losing weight. Instead, it will make the fast last just long enough that you will be able to speed up the metabolism.

With the intermittent fast, you will find that when you go for a few hours without eating (usually no more than 24ish hours), the body is not going to go right into starvation mode. Rather, it is going to consume the calories that are available. If you ate the right number of calories for the day, the body is going to revert to eating up the stored reserves of fat and use it as fuel. As such, when following an intermittent fasting plan, you force your body to burn more fat without putting in any extra work.

Here are few quick tips for success:

First and foremost, it is important to not expect to see results from your new lifestyle immediately. Instead, you need to plan on committing to the process for at least 30 days before you can start to accurately judge the results.

Second, it is important to keep in mind that the quality of the food you put into your body still matters as it will only take a few fast food meals to undo all of your hard work.

Finally, for the best results, you will want to add in a light exercise routine during fast days and a more traditional routine for full-calorie days.

Types of intermittent fasting

There are a few major types of intermittent fasting that you can choose to work with. These fasts can all be effective, and the one that's right for you will depend on your personal preferences, schedule, and lifestyle. Some of the fasting options that you can go with include:

- The 16/8 method: This one will ask you to fast for 16 hours each day and eat during the other 8 hours. So, you may choose to only eat from noon to 8 pm or from 10 am to 6 pm. You can choose whichever eight-hour window that you like.
- Eat-Stop-Eat: Once or twice each week, you will not eat anything from dinner one day until dinner the next day. This gives you a 24-hour fast but still allows you to eat on each of the days that you are fasting.
- The 5:2 diet: You will pick out two days of the week to fast. During those two days, you are only allowed to have up to 500-600 calories each day.

Of course, there are variations of the three that are listed above. For example, some people decide to limit their windows even more and only eat for four hours and fast for twenty on this diet. Most people who go on these fasts will choose to go with the 16/8 method because it's the easiest to stick with and will give you some great results in the process.

Intermittent fasting is simple and effective. It helps you limit the calories that you are consuming and burn more fat and calories than you would with a traditional diet.

Chapter 3: How Can I Fast?

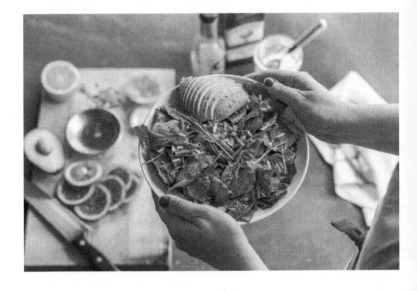

One thing that a lot of people like about intermittent fasting is that it provides you with a lot of choices. As mentioned, there are a few different ways that you can do an intermittent fast based on your schedule and lifestyle. Some people find that they have a few busy days during the week and so will fast on those days. Others like the idea of limiting their eating window and doing a small fast each day.

The fasting method that you choose is up to you. All of them can be effective and will provide you with some of the benefits that you are looking for. Let's take a look at some of the fasting options that you can go with, so you can choose the right one for you.

The 16/8 Method

This is one of the most common methods that you can use in intermittent fasting. It requires that you fast for about 14 to 16 hours each day and eat during the remainder of the hours. During this eating window, you are still able to fit in two to three meals without a problem. This is more likely to fit into the eating schedule that you are used to, but it still limits you so that you do not eat all day long.

This method is easier than you think. It is as easy as not eating any snacks after you are done with dinner and then skipping breakfast, or at least having a late breakfast. So, if you finish your last meal at 8 at night and then do not eat anything until noon the next day, you are already fasting for 16 hours. You just have to be careful about the late-night snacks. If you eat them, you will need to avoid breakfast in the morning.

Some people have issues with this because they feel hungry in the morning and feel they need to eat breakfast. You can simply move breakfast to a little later in the day. For example, if you choose to eat breakfast at 10 in the morning instead of 8 and then stop eating by 6 at night, you would still be within the 16-hour window.

If you're a woman, this is the option that you should probably go with. Women typically do the best with these shorter fasts and may want to consider going with 14 to 15 hours between eating because this is more effective for them.

During the fast, you are allowed to drink water, tea, coffee, and other beverages that are non-caloric to help reduce the hunger pains that occur. In addition, you should try to stick with healthier foods during your eating window. It is not a good idea to eat a lot of unhealthy food during this time. Some people like to go on a low-carb diet when they are on intermittent fast because it helps with hunger and allows for better results.

The 5:2 diet

Another option that you can go with is the 5:2 diet. This one asks you to eat normally for five days during the week and restrict yourself to no more than 600 calories on each of the other two days. This is sometimes called "the Fast diet" as well.

On these fasting days, it is recommended that women stay around 500 calories and men at 600 calories. For instance, you will eat normally each day of the week, and on Monday and Thursdays, you will only eat two small meals with a total of 500-600 calories. You can choose any days of the week as your fasting days, as long as you don't have them back to back. Pick your two busiest days of the week and make those your fasting days.

There are not many studies out there about the 5:2 diet, but since it is an intermittent fast, it will provide most of the benefits that you are looking for. You will be able to get things done without having to worry about making meals the whole day.

Eat-Stop-Eat diet

The Eat-Stop-Eat diet requires you to refrain from eating for 24 hours once or twice a week. This method was first popularized by Brad Pilon and has been a popular way to do the intermittent fast for some time. It's possible to follow this fast while still having one meal a day. Most people will have supper one day and then not eat anything until supper the next day. This allows you to never go a whole day without eating but still fall in the 24-hour abstinence period.

You can change this however you like. If it is easier for you to go from breakfast to breakfast or lunch to lunch, then you can choose one of these options. During your fast, you are allowed to have coffee, water, and other non-caloric beverages to keep yourself hydrated, but you're not allowed to have any food at all.

Remember that you are only fasting for one or two days a week. When it's time to eat normally, you need to eat the same amount of food that you would have if you were not on a fast. This will help you to lose weight without harming your body.

The biggest issue with going on this kind of intermittent fast is that fasting for 24 hours is hard for most people. However, you can ease into it. You may find that starting with a shorter fast, such as the 16-hour fast, can provide some good results and then can start fasting for longer periods of time. Going an entire day without eating can be tough, and most people choose to go with one of the other fasting options to see the same results.

Alternate day fasting

With this option, you will go on a fast every other day. There are a few options that you can go with, and it will depend on what works for your needs. Some of these fasts will allow you to have about 500 calories on your fasting days. You will find that most of the lab studies concerning intermittent fasting used some version of the alternate day fast to help determine all the health benefits.

Fasting every other day can be difficult for most people. Forcing yourself to fast every other day can be a challenge. Fasting every other day is something that you will probably need to build up to. You will likely feel really hungry several times a week on this fasting plan, and it is hard to stick with over the long-term.

Warrior Diet

This is another popular option that you can choose when it comes to intermittent fasting. It involves eating small amounts of raw fruits and vegetables during the day followed by a large meal at night. This requires you to fast all day, eating just enough to keep you satisfied, and then feasting at night within a four-hour eating window.

The warrior diet is one of the first diets to incorporate some form of intermittent fasting. The warrior diet also includes food choices that mimic the Paleo diet. You will not only fast during most of the day and feast at night, but you will eat a diet that is full of unprocessed foods that resemble what you can find out in nature.

Spontaneous Meal Skipping

You can try this if you want to prepare your body for intermittent fasting or if you don't want to spend much time worrying about when you can eat. With this fast, you do not need to worry about following one of the more structured intermittent fasting plans. You will just skip some meals from time to time. You can do this when you are not hungry or when you are just too busy to have a meal. It is a big myth that you have to eat something every few hours to avoid starvation.

The body is well adapted to handle long periods of time without eating. Missing out on a few meals, especially if you are not hungry or too busy, is not harmful to your body.

Any time you end up skipping a meal or two, you are technically fasting. If you are too busy to grab a breakfast on the way out the door, just make sure that you eat a healthy lunch and dinner. If you are out running errands and you are not able to find someplace to eat, then it is fine to miss out on a meal. This is not going to cause any harm and will actually help you save time.

You probably won't see as good of results compared to some of the other options, but it is better than nothing and is a lot easier to work with. Perhaps try to skip a meal or two during the week or miss some meals when it works for you.

As you can see, there are several different options that you can work with when you are ready to go on the intermittent fast. Some of these will be easier than others, and some may fit your schedule better. You will need to choose which fast is easiest for you to work within your daily life.

Chapter 4: Why Should I Try Intermittent Fasting?

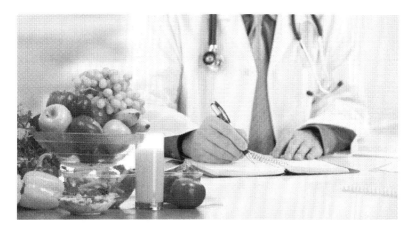

There are a lot of different diet plans that you can choose from. Some help you limit your carb intake and focus on the good fats and proteins. Some will limit your fat intake and focus on good and healthy carbs.

With all of the choices on the market, and with at least a few of them being legitimate options for losing weight, you may be curious as to why you should go with intermittent fasting. This chapter will take a look at the various benefits of intermittent fasting and how it will make a difference in your health.

Changes the function of hormones, genes, and cells

When you do not eat for some time, several things happen to your body. For example, your body will start initiating processes for cell repair and change some of your hormone levels, which makes stored body fat easier to access. Other changes that can happen in the body include:

- Insulin levels: Your insulin levels will drop by quite a bit, which makes it easier for the body to burn fat.
- Human growth hormone: The blood levels of the growth hormone can greatly increase. Higher levels of this hormone can help build muscle and burn fat.
- Cellular repair: The body will start important cellular repair processes, such as removing all the waste from cells.
- Gene expression: Some beneficial changes occur in several genes that will help you to live longer and protect against disease.

Lose weight and body fat

Many people go on an intermittent fast to lose weight. In most cases, intermittent fasting will naturally help you to eat fewer meals. You will end up taking in fewer calories, which will lead to weight loss.

In addition, fasting enhances the hormone function to facilitate weight loss. Higher growth hormone levels and lower insulin help your body to break down fat and use it for energy. This is why short-term fasting can increase your metabolism by at least three percent.

On one side, it boosts your metabolic rate so that you burn more calories while also reducing how much you eat. According to a 2014 review of scientific research on intermittent fasting, people were able to lose up to 8 percent of their body weight in less than 24 weeks.

Helps with diabetes

Type-2 diabetes is a disease that has become widespread in recent decades. Anything that reduces your insulin resistance should help lower your blood sugar levels and protect you against type 2 diabetes. Some studies show how intermittent fasting can have benefit in insulin resistance and can help lead to a dramatic reduction in blood sugar levels.

In several studies on intermittent fasting, blood sugar was reduced by three to six percent, while insulin was reduced by twenty to thirty-one percent. One study on diabetic rats also showed that intermittent fasting was able to protect the rat against kidney damage, which is a common complication with more serious forms of diabetes. This shows that intermittent fasting may be a good option for anyone with a higher risk of developing type 2 diabetes.

There are some differences between the genders. There is one study that showed that for women, blood sugar control could actually get worse after going on the intermittent fast for a few weeks. It's recommended to talk to your physician before starting any kind of diet plan.

Simplifies life

While this may not be considered a health benefit like the others, it is still an important one to mention. Many people find that intermittent fasting can make their lives easier. They find that they do not need to focus too much on the calories they are eating, as long as they stay within the hours that they are allowed to eat. They can go a few days a week without having to worry about making a meal. Overall, this diet plan can make your life easier.

When you can cut out some of the work that you need to do during the day and focus on something else, you can end up with less stress in your life. We all know how too much stress can have a negative impact on our health and life. When you can reduce stress, it is much easier to be the healthiest version of yourself.

Good for the heart

Heart disease is considered one of the biggest killers in the world. Intermittent fasting can help with some of these risk factors, such as lowering blood sugar levels, inflammatory markers, blood triglycerides, cholesterol, and blood pressure.

The biggest issue is that a lot of studies on intermittent fasting have been done on animals. We need to have more studies that test intermittent fasting and heart health in humans.

Can help with cancer

Many people suffer from cancer each year. This terrible disease is characterized by uncontrolled growth of cells. Fasting has been shown to have some great benefits when it comes to your metabolism, which could lead to a reduced risk of cancer.

Some human studies show that cancer patients who fasted were able to reduce some of the side effects that come with chemotherapy.

Good for the brain

What is considered good for the body is good for the brain as well. Intermittent fasting can help improve metabolic features that are known for helping the brain to stay healthy as well. This could include helping with insulin resistance, blood sugar level reduction, reduced inflammation and oxidative stress.

There have been several studies done on rats that show how intermittent fasting can help increase the growth of new nerve cells, which improves the brain's function. Fasting can also help to increase the levels of the brain-derived neurotrophic factor. When the brain is deficient in this, it can cause depression as well as some other brain issues.

Helps with cellular repair

When we go on a fast, the cells in the body can initiate a waste removal process that is known as autophagy. This involves the cells breaking down and metabolizing any proteins that can't be used any longer. With an increased amount of autophagy, it could help protect the body against diseases such as Alzheimer's and cancer.

May prevent Alzheimer's

Alzheimer's is one of the most common neurodegenerative diseases. There is no cure for Alzheimer's, so your best course of action is to prevent it from happening. One study that was done on rats showed that intermittent fasting might be able to delay the onset of Alzheimer's disease, or at least reduce the severity of it.

Some case reports have shown that a lifestyle alteration that included some daily, or at least frequent, short-term fasts helped to improve the symptoms of Alzheimer's in 9 out of 10 patients. Animal studies also show that this kind of fasting could help to protect against other neurodegenerative diseases, such as Huntington's disease and Parkinson's.

While most of these studies have been done on animals, the results look promising. Intermittent fasting is a trend, and studies on ways it makes your body healthier are relatively new. It will take some time to study all the benefits of intermittent fasting.

Intermittent fasting could help you to live longer

One of the most exciting things about intermittent fasting is that it can help you live longer. There have been several studies of rats that showed how intermittent fasting could help extend their lifespan - similar to what happens when you go on a continuous calorie restriction. In some of the studies, the effects were dramatic. In one of them, when the rats fasted every other day, they ended up living 83 percent longer than the rats who didn't do fasting.

Although it has been hard to prove an increase in lifespan because intermittent fasting has yet to be studied on people long enough to determine this, it is still a popular idea for those who are trying to prevent aging. Given that there are known benefits to metabolism with this diet, it is no wonder that people believe that intermittent fasting will able to help them live longer and healthier lives.

As you can see, there are lots of benefits of going with the intermittent fasting diet. We only touched on a few of them, but there have been many studies done on the effects of this diet and why it can benefit you. Whether you are trying to improve brain health, live longer, lose weight, or get more energy, intermittent fasting can improve your life.

Chapter 5: Fasting, Training, and Eating

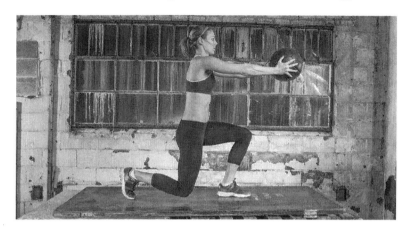

A lot of people will see results with intermittent fasting on its own. They do a good job of eating during certain windows, and when they eat, they make sure that their food is full of nutrition. But if you would like to enhance your results and burn extra fat, then it is important to add some workouts to your routine. This chapter will take a look at the steps that you should take to properly train and exercise while on the intermittent fast.

In fact, a study recently conducted by a Sport and Health Sciences institute in Sweden shows that reducing the overall number of carbs in your diet allows your body to burn calories more effectively and increase muscle growth potential. In this study, ten elite level cyclists went through an hour of interval training, going at about 64 percent of their maximal aerobic capacity. They either had low or normal muscle glycogen levels that were achieved before diet or exercise intervention.

Ten muscle biopsies were taken before exercise, as well as three hours after they were done with exercising. The results showed that exercising while in a glycogen depleted state was able to increase mitochondrial biogenesis. This is the process by which new mitochondria can form inside the cells. The authors of the study believe that exercising on a low glycogen level diet may be beneficial for improving muscle oxidative capacity.

Part of what makes working out when you are currently in a fasted state effective is that the body has some mechanisms that help to preserve and protect the muscles from wasting itself. So, if you are low on fuel for a workout, which you naturally will be when you are on an intermittent fast, your body will start to break down some of the other tissues, but not the active muscle that you're using.

Exercising while preserving your muscles

Many experts agree that about 80% of the health benefits that you gain from a healthy lifestyle comes from your diet. The rest will come from exercise. This means that you need to focus on eating the right foods if you want to actually lose weight. However, it is important to realize that both exercise and eating well are necessary.

Researchers studied the data from 11 participants who were on the show "The Biggest Loser." The total body fat, total energy expenditure, and the resting metabolic rate of the participants were measured three times. These were measured at the start of the program, after six weeks, and then at 30 weeks. Using a model of the human metabolism, the researchers were able to calculate the impact of diet and exercise changes in resulting in weight loss to see how each one contributed to this goal.

Researchers found that the diet alone was responsible for most of the weight loss. However, only about 65 percent of that weight loss was from body fat. The rest of the reduction in body weight was from lean muscle mass. Exercise alone resulted in fat loss only, along with a slight increase in lean muscle mass.

According to the National Institutes of Health, *"The simulations also suggest that the participants could sustain their weight loss and avoid weight regain by adopting more moderate lifestyle changes – like 20 minutes of vigorous daily exercise and 20 percent calorie restriction – than those demonstrated on the television program."*

Exercising and fasting together

If you are trying to get an effective exercise program that will add some high-intensity training as well as intermittent fasting, there are a few components that will need to come together. When you are doing this, if you feel that you do not have enough energy to keep going with the workouts, then it is time to make a change. Usually reducing how many hours you are fasting for will make a difference. Intermittent fasting is meant to make you feel great, and if it doesn't, then it is time to change up your strategy.

There are two main points that you need to keep in mind when working out while on the intermittent fast. The first one is about the timing of your meals. Intermittent fasting is not all about extreme calorie restrictions. You are not meant to starve yourself to achieve great results. Rather, it is simply a matter of timing your meals properly so that you do not eat during most of the day. You can eat during a small window, perhaps during the evening or later part of the day. So, if you limit your eating to between 4 and 7 in the evening, you will be fasting for 21 hours.

It is ideal for most people to go between 12 to 18 hours of fasting. Most people prefer to fast for 16 hours because this is the easiest to fit into their busy schedules. You can find out what works the best for your needs while ensuring that you will get all of the benefits.

If you are having trouble completely abstaining from food during the day, then you want to limit your eating to a small serving of light, low-glycemic foods. These include healthy options like poached eggs, whey protein, vegetables, and fruits every four to six hours. Whatever times you decide to eat, it's best to avoid food at least three hours before you go to bed. Doing this will help you minimize the oxidative damage in your system and can really make intermittent fasting easier to accomplish.

In addition, you should break your fasts with a recovery meal on the days that you work out. On the days that you have to exercise while fasting, you need to consume a recovery meal about 30 minutes after you're done working out. Adding fast-assimilating whey protein to your meal can help with muscle recovery.

After you have had that meal, it's a good idea to fast again until you eat your main meal that night. It's important to eat an appropriate recovery meal after each workout session. This will ensure that your body gets the energy that it needs, and that muscle or brain damage will not occur. Do not skip this meal and make sure that you are getting it within 30 minutes after the workout.

If you think that fasting for 12 to 18 hours is difficult to accomplish, it is possible to get the same benefits from exercise and fasting by skipping breakfast and exercising right away in the morning when you have an empty stomach. This is because eating a big meal before a workout, especially one that is carb-heavy, inhibits the sympathetic nervous system and reduces the fat burning effects of your exercise.

While most people have been taught that they need to take in a lot of carbs before a workout to get endurance and see results, this works against the goals that you have. Eating too many carbs activates the parasympathetic nervous system that promotes energy storage and stores calories and carbs inside the body. This is likely the last thing that you want if you are exercising and on the intermittent fast, so it's best to fast to see better results.

Tips for getting the most out of your workouts

Working out on an intermittent fast is not meant to be hard. Exercise and plenty of physical movement are meant to help you feel good, build muscle and lose more weight. Some of the ways that you can make sure you really do well when working out on an intermittent fast include:

- Start out slow—if you have never done a weightlifting program before, you will need to start out slowly. Even if you are just returning to an existing exercise routine, it is important to remember the changes you have made and take it slow until you know how they will affect your performance.

- Add more weight when you feel comfortable—it is important to consistently add on more weights when you start to feel comfortable. Over time, the weights that you begin your workout with will start to feel pretty light, and if you don't make some changes, you will find that your results will slow down. This doesn't mean you want to force your body past its limits, but it does mean you will want to regularly increase the difficulty of your exercise routine if you hope to see continued success.

- Fewer reps and more weight is best for lean muscles- If you are looking to build lean muscle, consider doing fewer repetitions at a higher weight. This can exhaust the body faster and will give you better results.

- Don't forget to warmup and cool down – Just because you have to change your eating habits doesn't give you an excuse to cut out the warmup and cooldown portions of your exercise routine. Taking at least five minutes at the start and conclusion of the workout to stretch your muscles will not only improve performance, it will reduce the likelihood of injury as well.

- Focus on form—sometimes we get too focused on how much weight we can lift when working out at the gym. However, having proper form is actually more important. It is better to do an exercise with the right form with lower weight than to add on more weight and do it poorly.

Chapter 6: The Basics of Eating on an Intermittent Fast

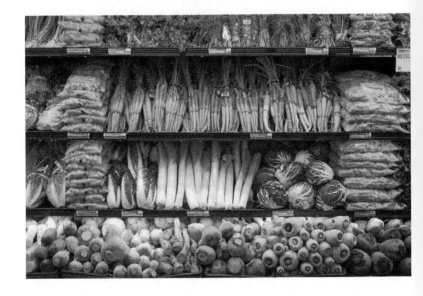

Eating on the intermittent fast can be as simple or as complicated as you choose. Some people will continue with their healthy eating ahead of time and others who will add another type of diet to this one to see results. The ketogenic diet can work pretty well with this option because it helps to limit your carbs to reduce hunger and to burn the fat more quickly.

However, it's not essential for you to go on a specific diet plan to see results when on an intermittent fast.

The first thing to keep in mind is that you are not allowed to eat unhealthy food when you are on this kind of diet plan. It is good to cut down your window of eating during the day to eight hours or less (or to do one of the other options for intermittent fasting). But, if you spend that time eating desserts, fast foods, and other unhealthy foods, you will run into problems.

First, you will not be able to lose weight when you eat this way. Fast foods and other unhealthy choices come with many calories per serving, and it's likely that you are taking in more than one serving at a time. Even though your window for eating is smaller, you can still take in too many calories, which will stop all your weight loss progress. Even though intermittent fasting is not about the calorie-intake, you still need to be cautious about eating too many calories because it's an aspect that can affect the effectiveness of intermittent fasting.

You will also notice that when you eat these unhealthy foods, even while on an intermittent fast, you will not improve your health. Your health will rely on good food that is high in nutrients to keep you strong. Simply fasting, while still eating unhealthy food, will likely cause as many problems as you encountered before you started fasting.

When you eat these bad food, you will find that you are hungry more often and you will struggle with getting through your fasting periods. This is because many processed and fast foods contain chemicals and preservatives that are designed to make you hungry more often. If you want to see the results and get through your fast without feeling hungry, then it is time to eat foods that are healthier.

Now, this doesn't mean that you can't eat sweets or junk food on occasion. The intermittent fast doesn't have set rules for exactly what you are allowed to eat, it simply sets the times that you are allowed to eat. Eating a little cheat meal is fine, as long as you have it during your eating windows and only do it on occasion. It may be hard sometimes but eating healthier will provide you with better results.

The trick to making the intermittent fast work for you is to eat a healthy diet. The more nutrients you can fit into your diet plan, the better you will end up doing with this fast.

The first thing that you need to consider is eating plenty of fruits and vegetables. Fresh produce is best because it provides lots of essential nutrients that your body needs to stay healthy. Consider filing your plate with fruits and vegetables each meal so that you are getting the nutrients that you need. Eating a wide variety of produce is also important to ensure that you are getting what your body needs without adding in too many calories.

Next, you should go with some good sources of protein. You should consider going with options like lean ground beef, turkey, and chicken. Having some bacon and other fatty meats on occasion is fine, just don't overdo it. Eating a lot of fish will help you to get the healthy fatty acids that the body needs to function properly.

Healthy sources of dairy help you to stay lean while giving your body the calcium it needs. You can have some options such as milk, yogurt (be careful of the kinds that have fruit and other things added because these usually include a high amount of sugar), sour cream, cheese, etc. Be sure to monitor the salts and sugars that are not healthy for the body.

You are allowed to have some carbs on this diet. Carbs have gotten a bit of a bad reputation because so many diet plans recommend that you avoid them. The important thing here is to eat the carbs that are healthy for you. White bread and pasta are basically sugars in disguise and should be avoided. Going with whole grain and whole wheat options when it comes to your carbs will ensure that you can get all the nutrition that you need.

Having a well-balanced diet will be the key to ensuring that you feel good when you are on an intermittent fast. You will be able to mix up the meals that you choose, so you get the best results when you go on this kind of a fast.

You are also allowed to have a snack, as long as you are careful with how often this happens. If you are eating junk, you will be disappointed when you go to the scale and see that you are not losing weight. You can have treats on occasion, but make sure that it is not something that you often while on this diet.

Using the ketogenic diet with intermittent fasting

Lots of people decide to go on a ketogenic diet while doing an intermittent fast to help stay healthy. The ketogenic diet is a high fat, moderate protein, and low carb diet that will help you to burn fat quickly while reducing your dependence on carbs. There is a lot to love with this diet plan, and when it is combined with the intermittent fasting, you are sure to get some great results in no time.

It's possible to use both of these diet plans together. Intermittent fasting is focused on the times of day when you will eat, and the ketogenic diet on what to eat during those time periods. For those who would like to balance their blood sugar level and want to lose weight more efficiently, combining these two diet plans together can be great.

With intermittent fasting, you limit the hours that you can eat. Instead of spreading your meals and your snacks throughout the day, you will limit it to just a few hours. Many people will choose to only eat between ten and six and fit their macronutrients into that time period. Others will take two or three days during the week where they are not allowed to eat and fit their nutrients into the other days of the week.

The point is that you are limiting the amount of time that you eat, forcing you to think more about the foods you consume. You also get the benefit of more fat burning and weight loss, when you do intermittent fasting.

During the times you are allowed to eat, you will need to stick with the macronutrients that we discussed above that are approved for the ketogenic diet. You will still stick with high fat, moderate protein, and low carb diet plan even while intermittent fasting. You will just need to be more careful about the times you eat those macronutrients, but otherwise, you can follow the ketogenic diet exactly the same.

If you want to get some of the benefits of intermittent fasting or you want to increase your weight loss, then adding this diet in with the ketogenic diet can be effective. You can experiment with the different types of intermittent fasting options that are available to see which one fits into your schedule the best or works the best for you. Of course, if you find the ketogenic diet is effective or intermittent fasting is too difficult, you can always just stick with the ketogenic diet and not fast and still see good results.

It is important to remember that you don't have to follow the ketogenic diet if you don't want to while on an intermittent fast. Many people go choose other healthy diets instead of choosing to go on the ketogenic diet. However, there are a lot of people who will choose to go with the ketogenic diet along with intermittent fasting because it is easy to follow and will allow them to lose even more fat.

Eating on the intermittent fast does not need to be too difficult. You can pick out the foods that you want to eat, although it is important to go with foods that are fresh and whole and will fill you up and help with the fat burning process to help you to see the weight loss that you are looking for.

Chapter 7: Basic Tips for Intermittent Fasting

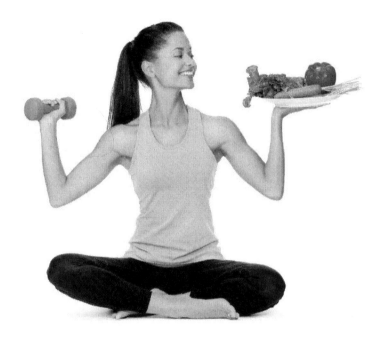

Getting started with intermittent fasting can take some time. You will have to change some of the eating patterns that you are used to, but it can be effective for you in so many ways. You will see that it is easier to lose weight, improve your energy, burn body fat, get more done, and protect against diseases such as diabetes, cancer, and dementia.

Although intermittent fasting is easier than most other diet plans out there, it still takes some work. Some of the things to keep in mind to get the most out of your intermittent fast are:

- Drink plenty of water: Water keeps you hydrated and makes you feel fuller when you are on your fast. Being in a fasted state also acts as a diuretic, which means that your body will naturally expel water at a faster rate than you are used to. What it all boils down to is that you are going to want to aim to consume a gallon of water a day for the best results.

- Drink tea and coffee: When you are feeling hungry, you may find that it's helpful to drink tea or coffee to keep down your appetite. Caffeine is a natural appetite suppressant. Just try not to consume any caffeine too close to bedtime (at least 3 hours), or you may have trouble falling asleep.

- Keep yourself busy: You may find that are more productive on an empty stomach. If you are keeping yourself busy, not only will you get more done, but you'll be able to distract yourself from the hunger. If you don't find productive ways to fill your time, especially at first, then you will find that the hours you are fasting seem to stretch out into days. Don't make things harder on yourself than they need to be. When it comes to the early days of your new eating habit, make sure your days are packed full of activities.

- Make it flexible: There are so many options that come with intermittent fasting. You do not have to go with one option because everyone else is. You can mix and match and create the schedule that works for you. Intermittent fasting is all about having the freedom to do it the way that you want.

- Try it for at least a month: You need at least three to four weeks to determine if the intermittent fast is right for you. If you don't do it for this long, then you are not giving the body the time it needs to adapt, and you are not giving it a fair shot. Try it out for at least this amount of time to see if it's the right choice for you.

- Experiment with fasting methods: What works for one person may not work for you. If you find that certain fasting times are better or that a particular version of intermittent fasting is more effective, then choose those. It's all experimenting to see what feels right for you.

- Delay your breakfast slowly: One thing that works well for a lot of people is to slowly delay their breakfast. By gradually pushing back your breakfast time an hour every week or so, you will eventually get yourself into an intermittent fast without it being too difficult. For instance, if you usually eat breakfast at 8 am, wait until 8:30 am to eat your breakfast for the first week. Then push your breakfast back to 9 am in week 2. Continue this process until your first meal occurs around noon.

- Drink water in the morning: Often the reason that you feel so hungry in the morning is that you have gone all night without eating. A good habit to start is to drink a glass of water right when you wake up in the morning.

- Add weights: If you are trying to lose weight and tone up, it makes sense to add some weight training to your routine. While you won't want to mix things up too much when you are first getting started, once your body has adapted to an intermittent fasting lifestyle, there is no reason you shouldn't take things up a notch. You will be surprised what your body can handle. If you take things slowly, eventually you should be able to handle a full-intensity workout without feeling too drained to function when you are finished.

- Live it up: With intermittent fasting, you need to realize that you can live it up on occasion. You can have fun as long as you ensure it all balances out in the end. While the average diet is all about the foods that you aren't allowed to eat, an intermittent fasting lifestyle accounts for the fact that sometimes you can't plan your meals. This means that as long as you get your fasting period in, there is no reason you can't move your hours around, as long as you don't do so constantly. What's more, there is no reason you can't indulge now and then, as long as one delicious and decadent dessert doesn't end up turning into seven or eight.

- Get out of the house: There is a lot of temptation in your home. Therefore, it is better to get out of the house, so you don't eat all of that food. Even if you have kids around, think of an activity you all can do to keep yourselves occupied.

- Eat more protein and healthy fat: Eating additional protein with each meal makes it easier to control your appetite and build up your muscles. Eating more healthy fat will give you extra energy and help you feel fuller longer as well. Thanks to the insidious advancement of the Standard American Diet, a vast majority of those in the Western world eat far too many carbohydrates and not nearly enough protein or healthy fat. To rectify this problem, start considering the macros of the foods you eat. Also, ensure that when you are in an eating window you fill your plate with foods that will make sticking it out to the next window as easy as possible.

- Avoid the bad stuff: You need to make sure that you are not using it as an excuse to eat junk food all the time. Make sure to stick with a well-balanced diet so that you provide your body with enough nutrition, even if you choose to go on a fast. It is important to keep in mind that a big part of intermittent fasting is building up a calorie deficit by the end of the week to support additional weight loss. As such, if you fill your body full of high-calorie junk food when you do enter an eating window, what you are really doing is undoing all of your hard work. Making healthy choices at all times will improve the overall effectiveness of your weight loss efforts, guaranteed.

As you can see, there are a lot of different things you can do to get the most out of intermittent fasting. This doesn't mean you should expect constant weight loss, however, regardless of how strict your fasting might be. While you will likely see weight loss at first as your body adapts to fewer calories in its system; this will likely start and stop throughout your time fasting. The effects are especially noticeable after the first few weeks of the transition as your body tries to hold on to everything it has until it can figure out what is going on. Once it gets with the program, however, things should proceed as expected.

Every diet is going to have periods of weight loss plateau. That is simply a part of weight loss that cannot be mitigated. As long as you stay consistent, weight loss will eventually resume. The worst thing you can do is to try and change things up to get weight loss back on track as that will only make it more difficult for your body to start losing weight again. Instead, if you stay the course and keep up the good work, you will start seeing results again before you know it.

Chapter 8: Intermittent Fast FAQs

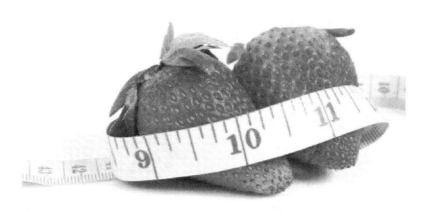

There are a lot of questions that you may have with intermittent fasting. You want to make sure that you are doing it the right way and that you will be able to get all the benefits that are promised with this diet plan. This chapter will take some time to explore more about intermittent fasting and what you need to know to get it to work for you.

Is there anyone who shouldn't fast?

For the most part, intermittent fasting is safe for most people to do. It's an effective diet plan that focuses on healthy eating and getting the essential calories and nutrition that your body needs while restricting the windows that you're allowed to eat.

With that said, some people should not go on an intermittent fast. This is mostly because there is concern that they will not be able to get the nutrition that they need. If you're considered underweight, you should not go on this kind of fast. If you're pregnant or breastfeeding, you need to take in nutrients throughout the day to support your child, so intermittent fasting is not the option for you.

In addition, there are times when you are allowed to fast, but you may want to make sure that you have some supervision from your doctor. First, if you have diabetes, either type 1 or type 2, you will need to do this with the help of your doctor. Some medications don't work well with these fasts so you will need to be careful. In addition, if you have high uric acid or gout, you may need to be careful about going on an intermittent fast.

Will I go into starvation mode if I am fasting?

There are a lot of myths about fasting. These myths are repeated so often that sometimes they are seen as truths. Some of the fasting myths that you may know about include:

- Fasting makes you starve
- Fasting will you feel hungry
- Fasting will make you overeat when the fast is over
- Fasting will make you lose muscle tone

These have been disproven many times over. Instead of the body going into starvation mode, the body will start burning up the extra fat stored inside. This will help you to get rid of that stubborn belly fat and will help you become healthier, especially if you have been overeating for a long time.

Over a year, you consume about 1000 meals and over 60 years, you will eat about 60,000 meals. To say that skipping three meals during this time will cause a lot of harm is kind of silly.

The breakdown of muscle tissue only occurs at low levels of body fat, and if you are at that point, then you shouldn't go on a fast. However, most people will not have this issue. Our bodies are actually evolved to handle periods of starvation and will be able to effectively deal with it.

What are some side effects of going on a fast?

There are a few side effects that you can deal with when you are on a fast. These are usually pretty simple, and they will go away after your body adjusts to the diet and you get familiar with eating habits that work well. Some of the side effects that you may experience include:

- Constipation: This is a common side effect. If you're experiencing constipation, using some laxatives can to help to alleviate the pain or discomfort.

- Headaches: Some people experience headaches when they get started on a fast, but these will disappear within a few days. A good way to deal with this is to eat some extra salt each day.
- Mineral water: If you are dealing with your stomach gurgling, then it is a good idea to use mineral water.
- Other side effects: You may also deal with issues such as muscle cramps, dizziness, and heartburn. Adjusting your diet and waiting a few days will help to alleviate any discomfort.

How do I manage hunger?

The most important thing to realize is that this hunger will pass. Most people worry that the hunger will keep growing until it is intolerable, but this usually isn't the case. Hunger comes in waves. Ignoring it and drinking some water, tea, or coffee will help you to cope with the hunger pains.

During your extended fast, you might notice that the hunger will increase into the second day. After you get past that time, you will see that it recedes, with many people reporting that they have a complete loss of hunger by day 3 or 4. At this time, your body is powered by fat. This means that the body is eating its own fat for breakfast, lunch, and dinner, so you are no longer feeling so hungry. So, if you can last a few days on the intermittent fast, the hunger pains will go away, and it will be easier to deal with.

It is important to keep in mind that when you are first starting out your body is likely to struggle with fasting because it is used to have ready access to fuel all the time. Most of us are used to eating, even when we are not hungry, and the body will fight against your new habit with extreme hunger pains in an effort to get back on track. However, whether you go with the 16/8 fast, the 5:2 fast, or the alternate day fast, the truth of the matter is that you are not putting your body through anything it cannot handle. As such, as long as you stay the course, things will likely settle down in about a week or so once your body realizes that it is not, in fact, starving.

In order to make the transition as manageable as possible, the first thing you are going to want to do is to add more caffeine to your diet. While not acceptable in the long-term, this is a great way to keep the worst of the hunger pains away when they are at their sharpest. Additionally, you will want to ensure that your schedule is full during this time as the more activity your mind has to focus on, the faster time will fly. Finally, if you are already committed to an exercise plan, then you will want to ensure that you exercise right before you break your fast so that your body will get the fuel it needs to make the most of your efforts.

Will my fasting burn muscle?

This is a common misconception that a lot of people deal with when they are considering an intermittent fast. During the fasting periods, the body is first going to break down the glycogen into glucose so that it can be used for energy. After the glucose is all gone, the body will increase how much fat it's breaking down and use that for energy. Excess amino acids, which are the building blocks of protein, can also be used for energy. However, the body is not going to use its own muscle as fuel unless you're not eating for weeks on end.

Fasting is a practice that has been done for thousands of years. It's safe and effective, and unless you go for weeks without eating (and none of the intermittent fasting options ask you to fast for more than 24 hours), there is no reason to worry about losing excess muscle.

How do I break the fast?

Breaking the fast is one of the hardest parts of this diet and is likely the true test of whether or not you will be able to sustain it in the long-term. When you break your fast it is important to do so in moderation for multiple reasons. First, it is important to not add too much to your system all at once as this can put stress on your body and damage your stomach and intestines if repeated too often. Additionally, if you allow yourself to gorge when your resolve is at its weakest then you are far more likely to overeat and undue all the hard work you have done by fasting in the first place.

The best way to ensure that this does not happen is to plan ahead. Prepare the meal while you are waiting for the fast to end and ensure that it has very clearly defined portions. A hearty omelet is a good choice as you can fill it full of healthy, filling items and you can't easily go back for seconds. Meanwhile, a full pot of oatmeal is a poor choice as you could easily go through it without thinking twice.

Can women fast?

Yes, women can fast. The only exception to this rule is if you're underweight, pregnant, or breastfeeding. This is because you need those extra nutrients and should not go so long without eating in these situations. Other than that, it is perfectly fine for women to fast. In addition, the average weight loss with fasting is the same for men and women so it can be effective for both genders.

Tips for intermittent fasting

Getting started with intermittent fasting can be a challenge at times. To summarize, tips you can follow include:

- Drink lots of water
- Stay busy
- Drink coffee or tea to suppress hunger
- Find a good support group who can help you
- Ride out the hunger waves because they will go away
- Try to go on a low-carb diet. This will help you with reducing hunger and can make fasting easier. It can also help out with more weight loss.
- Give it a month
- Break a fast gently
- Do not binge when you are done with fasting

Final Thoughts

Intermittent fasting is a great option if you want to burn fat, lose weight, and get in better shape. This diet is not only about the foods that you eat. It is about the time of the day that you eat these foods so that you can be healthy and get your body to do the hard work for you.

The hardest part of this diet is to teach yourself to not eat all the time. We have been taught that we need to eat five or six meals a day (which is fine if they're small meals), but this isn't the case for most people. With intermittent fasting, you will be able to get the results that you need without having to work so hard.

Intermittent fasting is not just a weight-loss diet. It aims for more than that. It has several health benefits that will not only make you slimmer but also healthier and disease-free.

Conclusion

Thanks for making it through to the end of this book. I hope it was informative and able to provide you with all of the tools you need to achieve your health and fitness goals.

The next step is to get started on your journey with intermittent fasting. Intermittent fasting offers many benefits for your body. Whether you are looking to lose weight or improve your health, intermittent fasting is the way to go.

There are also a lot of options that come with intermittent fasting so you can pick the option that will work the best for you. Intermittent fasting is simple, easy to work with, and effective. When you are ready to lose weight or improve your health, refer back to this guidebook to help you get started.

Appendix

Coming up with a proper meal plan you can follow on your fasting days can be challenging with an intermittent fast. Here are some great meal plans you can follow to help make the intermittent fast work better for you.

Fast Day plan 1

Breakfast: Quaker Oats sachet of porridge (40g) - 255 calories

Dinner: Beetroot and feta salad - 125 calories

- Beetroot (50g) - 13 calories

- Feta (30g) - 83 calories

- Spinach (60g) - 29 calories

- A squeeze of lemon - 0 calories

Snack: Sliced apple with 1 tbsp. of almond butter - 145

Total calorie count: 525

Fast Day plan 2

Breakfast: Sweet plums and yogurt - 145 calories

- 100g low-fat natural yogurt - 65 calories

- 2 plums - 60 calories

- 1 tsp of honey - 20 calories

Dinner: Ryvita and tuna slices - 253 calories

- 2 x original Ryvita crackerbreads - 70 calories

- Tuna mayo (60g) - 171 calories

- Rocket (70g) sprinkled on top - 12 calories

- cracked black pepper - 0 calories

Snack: Miso soup - 32 calories

Total calorie count: 430

Fast Day plan 3

Breakfast: Soft boiled egg and asparagus - 90 calories

- 1 egg - 70 calories

- 5 pieces of asparagus - 20 calories

- salt and pepper to season

Dinner: Turkey burgers with corn-on-the-cob - 328 calories

- Minced turkey with beaten small egg, spring onion, garlic and chili (111g) - 172 calories

- 1 x corn-on-the-cob - 156 calories

Snack: A few frozen grapes - 60 calories

Total calorie count: 478 calories

Fast Day plan 4

Breakfast: Packet of Belvita Breakfast Biscuits (muesli) - 228 calories

Dinner: Roasted vegetables with balsamic glaze - 261 calories

- ½ courgette, ½ aubergine, ½ butternut squash, ½ red pepper - 247

- 1 tbsp. balsamic vinegar - 14 calories

- A squeeze of lemon - 0 calories

Snack: Harley's sugar-free jelly pot - 4 calories

Total calorie count: 493

Fast Day plan 5

Breakfast: spinach omelet - 160

- 2 x eggs - 140

- Spinach leaves (60g) - 20

- Salt and pepper - no calories

Dinner: Hummus and crudites - 175 calories

- Hummus (40g) - 123 calories

- A medium bowl full of carrots, cucumber, raw pepper - 52 calories

Snack: Edamame beans (60g) and rock salt - 84 calories

Total calorie count: 419

Fast Day plan 6

Breakfast: Banana and low-fat yogurt - 177 calories

- 100g low-fat natural yogurt - 65 calories

- 1 x banana - 112 calories

- A sprinkle of cinnamon - no calories

Dinner: Turkey breasts with wilted spinach - 216 calories

- 1 x turkey breast steak (125g) - 175 calories

- 1 cup of spinach, cooked and seasoned with salt - 41 calories

Snack: 10g of popcorn - 59 calories

Total calorie count: 452

F a s t   D a y   p l a n   7

Breakfast: Apple, carrot and ginger smoothie - 107 calories

- 1 apple - 55 calories

- 1 carrot - 52

- raw ginger - no calories

Dinner: Pitta pizza - 178 calories

- Weight Watchers wholemeal pitta - 106 calories

- 25g Extra Light Philadelphia cheese - 40 calories

- 1 tomato - 32 calories

- Mixed herbs - no calories

- Salt and pepper - no calories

Snack: 100g blueberries and a handful of almonds - 137 calories

Total calorie count: 422

Fasting Resources

- https://www.psychologytoday.com/blog/food-junkie/201308/the-american-diet
- https://www.healthline.com/nutrition/what-is-intermittent-fasting#section4
- https://www.healthline.com/nutrition/intermittent-fasting-guide#modal-close
- https://www.sciencedirect.com/science/article/pii/S193152441400200X
- http://ibimapublishing.com/articles/ENDO/2014/459119/
- https://www.ncbi.nlm.nih.gov/pmc/articles/PMC3946160/
- https://www.ncbi.nlm.nih.gov/pmc/articles/PMC3106288/
- https://www.ncbi.nlm.nih.gov/pubmed/25540982
- https://www.ncbi.nlm.nih.gov/pubmed/2405717
- https://www.karger.com/Article/Abstract/212538
- http://www.aging-us.com/article/100690

- https://www.ncbi.nlm.nih.gov/pubmed/17306982
- https://fitness.mercola.com/sites/fitness/archive/2012/11/02/interval-training-and-intermittent-fasting.aspx
- http://www.thefatlossninja.com/top-17-intermittent-fasting-tricks/

Book 2:

The Ultimate Fasting Diet:
Simple Intermittent Fasting Strategies to Boost Weight Loss, Control Hunger, Fight Disease, and Slow Down Aging

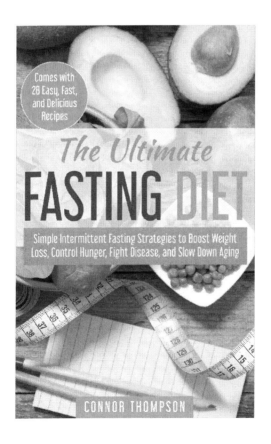

Introduction

Congratulations and thank you for downloading this eBook.

The following chapters will discuss everything that you need to know to get started and find success with intermittent fasting. There are a lot of diet plans on the market, however, many of these will not be effective. With intermittent fasting, you will be able to stick with this diet for a long time. There are a few options, so you can go with the method that ultimately works best for you.

In this guidebook, we are going to talk about intermittent fasting and how it can work for you. We will look at the basics of the fasting method including what it is, why so many people enjoy it, and more. We will also look at easy, delicious recipes that you can use on fasting days and non-fasting days. With this guidebook, you will understand exactly what you need to do to lose weight.

Other diet plans may be difficult to follow but going on an intermittent fast can be easy. Make sure that you read through this guidebook so you can start seeing great results with little effort.

There are plenty of books on this subject on the market; thanks again for choosing this one! It's my wish to provide you with the tools you need to make your dieting goals a success.

Chapter 1: Why Most Diets Don't Work

Most people have been on a diet at some point in their life for a variety of reasons. Maybe they wanted to lose a few pounds before going on a trip or vacation; maybe they tried to lose weight to feel better about themselves but got tired, bored, and gave up on the diet; or, maybe they just wanted to look their best for their high school reunion. No matter what the reason, it's likely that the diet only worked for a short period of time. Many diet plans are too hard to stick with long term, and when a diet is too hard to follow, the tendency is to give up and revert to old eating habits. Unsurprisingly, along with old eating habits, old weight is regained as well.

These diet plans (sometimes called yo-yo diets) are hard on the body. You want to lose weight and be healthy, however, most diet plans focus only on short-term results. More importantly, these diet plans often don't have an outline for how you can maintain the diet for the long term or they are too strict for the dieter to stick with for longer than a few months. There are many different types of diet plans for you to follow such as the Paleo Diet, the Low-Carb Diet, the Ketogenic diet, the vegetarian diet, and more. You can go on a diet plan that is going to restrict you from eating any fat and will ask you to focus on eating mostly fruits, vegetables, and a lot of carbs. Likewise, there are diet plans that will give you opposite advice and will tell you to dramatically reduce your carbs, and to instead focus on healthy fats and moderate amounts of protein. There are even diets on the market that have dieters go on a juice fast, cabbage soup diet, and other recommendations that are difficult to sustain.

While these diets can provide you with some short-term results, they are not good options if you are seeking long term results as they leave you hungry, possibly harm your body, and can even fuel negative thoughts about your self-image if you are unable to stick with the diet's unrealistic expectations. Along with these many diets, there is also a lot of conflicting advice that exists online. Think about how many times you have heard that fat is bad, and that carbs are good. However, the Ketogenic diet (which has become very popular) says the exact opposite: avoid carbs and eat more fat; this can be confusing for those who are looking to lose weight.

So, why do these diet plans ultimately fail? The main reason is that they are too strict or are too hard to follow; they are not designed for the typical person and how their busy schedule. They may have some good advice but being able to stick with them for a long period of time is quite difficult for most people. It can really hurt one's self-confidence when the diet is too demanding, and it's eventually abandoned. When it comes to weight loss, the goal should be changing your lifestyle rather than just changing the food that you consume. If you are someone who loves pasta, do you think you will be able to go on a low carb diet long term? If you are someone who loves a good steak or hamburger, do you think you will be able to stick to a vegetarian diet? Probably not.

Despite what other diet plans tell you, there is nothing wrong with eating these foods if you do so in moderation. Diets like the Ketogenic and Low-Carb diets spend too much time telling you what you are NOT allowed to eat so it becomes tedious to follow the strict guidelines every day. Of course, you want to follow the rules that come with your chosen diet. However, when you are told that you can't have something that you crave, no matter how hard you try, it's going to be that much more tempting to give in later.

This is why many people love intermittent fasting. While there are some recommendations in regard to which foods you should eat while on the intermittent fast, none of them are set in stone. You can still enjoy the foods you love as long as they are nutritious and if you eat them during the non-fasting phase of the diet. This makes it much easier for you to have the will power to stay on course during times of craving. If you can limit yourself to eating these foods during the non-fasting phase, you will see positive results in your weight loss.

The intermittent fast is about setting realistic, achievable goals that don't require superhuman willpower. This is a diet that you can get on and stay on because you can have variety in the things you eat so that it isn't a struggle every day. The hardest part of this diet is the first few days. While beginning the fasting phase, it's likely that you will experience hunger pains as your body isn't getting the same calorie intake that it's used to. However, with persistence, your body will adapt to these changes and the discomfort will pass. After you get over this hump, you will be well on your way to seeing excellent results!

With the help of the intermittent fasting diet, you will be able to break the cycle of dieting and relapse. With this diet, you will have the tools you need to get the results you are looking for. You will lose weight, have more energy throughout your day, and start to *feel* healthy again.

Chapter 2: The Science Behind Intermittent Fasting

The intermittent fasting diet is one of the best diet plans that you can adopt and it has a lot of great options to choose from. For example, you can choose to fast every day and limit the window of time that you allow yourself to eat during the day. Another option might be to fast for an entire day, or to choose specific days that you restrict your calories. Having these options makes it easier to adapt to your lifestyle because you have the flexibility to find the option that works best for you.

There are many types of fasts that you can choose from. Some people will choose to go with the 16/8 fast, which is one of the most common. This involves fasting for 16 hours of the day while being allowed to eat for the other 8 hours. Similarly, some people will allow themselves 10 hours to eat while others will allow for only 4 hours. There is some flexibility here that can suit your needs, so it's best to adjust the times you set aside to eat and to fast that best fit your life.

There are other options that you can go with as well, such as the 5:2 diet. This involves choosing 2 days a week where you can only eat up to 500 or 600 calories the whole day.

Another option is the warrior diet where you will fast all day and then feast on the last meal of the day. Some people will choose to fast for 24 hours between meals (such as going from supper one night to supper the next day).

These are just a few of the ways to do intermittent fasting and you can choose the one that works the best for your goals and needs.

The Benefits of the Intermittent Fast

There are many benefits when it comes to intermittent fasting. Some of the best reasons to choose an intermittent fast include:

- *Weight loss*: The main reason that a lot of people choose to go on an intermittent fast is to lose weight. This diet is great not only for losing weight, but also good at burning body fat as well.

- *Fights off cancer*: There are several studies done that show how the intermittent fast can help to fight off cancer or at least prevent it from occurring in the future. [Source 1][Source 2]

- *Boost your energy*: The intermittent fast can help you gain more energy than the typical American diet. Fat is a more efficient fuel source than carbs. This allows your body to provide you with more energy, so you can make it through the day.

- *Fights off heart disease*: Intermittent fasting can help to fight heart disease as well. As your body loses weight and burns fat, your blood pressure and cholesterol levels will decrease. This make things easier on your heart. [Source 1][Source 2]

- *Helps with diabetes*: Fasting helps you to burn through fat, rather than carbs. This can keep insulin levels low and helps to treat or prevent diabetes. There are many people who decide to go on an intermittent fast and combine it with a low-carb diet to help fight off diabetes. [Source 1][Source 2]

- *Keeps away Alzheimer's*: Intermittent fasting has been linked to preventing serious brain diseases, such as Parkinson's and Alzheimer's. This is good news for anyone worried about these diseases or anyone suffering from them already. [Source 1][Source 2]

- *Adds years to your life*: There have not been too many human studies on this yet, but many folks will argue that intermittent fasting helps you to live longer. If you are looking for a simple way to look and feel younger, then the intermittent fast may *be the right option for you*. [Source 1][Source 2]`

Facts About Intermittent Fasting

Although intermittent fasting provides many benefits, it does face some criticism. For instance, some people believe fasting to be unsafe because it deprives you of calories, makes you too hungry, or makes it harder to lose weight because your body goes into starvation mode. However, these are all myths as people have been fasting for centuries all over the world to stay healthy. As with any diet, you should consult with your doctor about your dieting plans and ensure that it's appropriate for you.

It Does NOT Include Binge Eating

Many critics claim that after a fast, dieters will indulge in overeating to try and regain "lost" calories. This is not true for most people. The goal of fasting is to learn how to control your eating habits so that you consume fewer calories and lose weight. While you may binge eat when hungry on other diets, with intermittent fasting, the goal is to fast and use self-control to remain disciplined. Remember, you can adjust the way you fast to cater to your needs. If you worry that you might struggle with this, fast for less time at the beginning and gradually increase it as you get more comfortable.

Starvation

The point of this diet is to train your brain to learn what your body actually needs. When fasting, you're not starving yourself – you are teaching your body that you can go without food for periods of time. Additionally, by gaining control over your eating habits you can prevent stress-eating, a common coping mechanism. When you have practiced intermittent fasting for a while, you will have a healthier approach to food and will be more likely to eat as a way to nourish your body rather than as a way to deal with your emotions.

Hard to Follow

In some cases, people worry that this diet will be hard to follow. This can be true during the first couple of days because you are working on changing the way that your body thinks about food. It (your body) will tell you to go get something sweet or to eat more to satisfy your cravings. However, once you become accustomed to the diet, it becomes easier because you will have control over your eating habits.

You Will Always be Hungry

There are going to be times when you will feel hungry when you first get started. Keep in mind that you just need to stick with it for a couple of weeks. Once that first week is done, it will be much easier. Eventually, you will have trained yourself to respond to hunger when it's time to eat, instead of as a reaction to cravings and hunger pains.

Intermittent fasting is not something that is impossible to follow and there are some basic principles to help guide you. For example, instead of trying to change everything about your diet from quantity to food selection, this diet instead focuses on changing *when* you eat while controlling your total calories.

Chapter 3: All About the Food

Eating on the intermittent fast does not have to be a challenge. In fact, other than making sure that you remain within your allotted calories, you can technically eat whatever you want and still see great results. With that said, as with most diets, you can't expect to see the same results when you are eating unhealthy foods like cookies, hotdogs, and other processed foods compared to other healthier options like fruits and vegetables.

Some people decide to incorporate other healthy diets with the intermittent fasting. If you are going to do this, it's recommended that you go with something like the ketogenic diet which is a high-fat, moderate protein, and low-carb diet will ensure that you are able to get good results because it will keep your body burning all that extra fat.

That said, it's important to realize that you do not need to go on a specific diet or follow a specific plan to see good results when it comes to the intermittent fasting diet. As long as you are able to stick with foods that are healthy and won't take up too many calories, you are going to see improved results for your body and health.

There are a few things that you need keep in mind when it comes to working with intermittent fasting. These are not hard-set rules that you must follow all the time, but they will allow you to eat the healthy foods that are necessary to ensure that you get the best results.

First, you need to make sure that you are eating plenty of quality produce. Fruits and vegetables will have great nutrients that your body needs and are great at curbing hunger without loading up on calories. You can eat plenty of these (apples, bananas, oranges, broccoli, tomatoes, etc.) even on those fasting days; just be sure to choose fresh ingredients as well as a variety of different fruits and veggies to make sure that you get the nutrients you need. If you're having a hard time coping with hunger, this is where you should turn to curb it.

Next, you need to make sure that you are consuming adequate amounts of protein while on your diet. This does not have to be a ton but adding in a little bit with each meal will keep your muscles strong, ensuring that you will keep yourself from feeling too hungry in the process. You should go for about 20 grams or more a day for women and 25 grams or more a day for men. There are a lot of great sources that you can use to help you get protein in your diet such as chicken, pork, ground beef, turkey, and fish.

Healthy fats are also allowed, you just have to be careful because there are major differences in the types of fats that you are able to eat. Saturated fats, like those found in most fast and processed foods, are not allowed on the intermittent fast. However, healthy fats such as fish and/or beef, or options like olive oil, will ensure that you are giving the body the fuel that it needs.

Some sources of dairy are fine as well such as milk, yogurt, cheese, and sour cream as they will ensure that your body is able to get the calcium that it needs to keep your muscles strong. These dairy sources can also be nice, low-fat sources of food that work well for snacks; however, you should be careful with dairy mixed with other types of food. Items to watch out for are yogurt with fruits or chocolate, strawberry milk, chocolate milk, etc. This is because many of these foods have added sugar, which takes away from their potential nutritional value.

Next, you need to watch the kinds of carbs that you are eating. If you are going on a diet plan like the ketogenic diet, then you will have to follow specific guidelines when it comes to the carbs that you can eat. However, if you are just going on an intermittent fast, you are fine with eating some carbs as long as you do not go crazy. Most women should stay under 150 carbs a day and men under 200 carbs a day. It's important to know the difference between the different carbs that you can consume.

First, you want to watch out for any processed carbs, white bread, and grains including baked goods, candies, processed foods, most fast foods. When these get into the body, they are treated the same as sugar, and this can cause a lot of trouble to your body as too many sugars and bad carbs could result in higher insulin levels which can lead to diabetes.

On the other hand, you can also work with whole grains because they are much healthier for you. This is primarily because they take longer to digest inside the body, which means that they will keep you fuller for longer. Grains are an important source of fiber, Vitamin B, thiamin, riboflavin, niacin, folate, as well as minerals like iron, magnesium, and selenium. They also have a lot of good nutrients that help to ensure that you stay healthy, even though you are going on a fast.

Other foods that are not on this list should be limited, but just because you are on a fast, it doesn't mean that you can't enjoy an occasional treat. Eating a snack after supper is not going to make much of a difference in the grand scheme of things, as long as you are careful to only indulge on occasion. Moderation is key when you work with this kind of fast.

As you can see, the rules for what you are allowed to eat when you are doing an intermittent fast are simple to work with. It's mostly a matter of making sure that you eat at the right time and that you stick to a decent calorie goal. When all of these are combined properly, you will start to see the weight loss and feel healthier

Chapter 4: Fasting vs. Non-Fasting Days

Now that you know a little bit about the foods that you can have while fasting, it's important to know how the different days during the fast work. This will make it easier for you to learn the rules of intermittent fasting so that you know what to expect when you are doing the fast.

The first thing to understand about this diet is the difference between fasting days and non-fasting days. Let's take a look at the fasting days first. The 5:2 fast allows you to eat during the fasting days but asks you to restrict your calories, you will need to limit your intake to 500 calories a day if you are a woman and 600 calories a day if you are a man; this is just enough to ensure that you get some good nutrition in, but not enough to stop your body from burning fat.

During fasting days, you can use your daily calorie allowance in whatever way you choose to spend it. For instance, some people choose to just go with one big meal because it helps them to splurge a bit when they are eating. When they're done, they don't have to fret over what they are going to eat for the rest of the day. Others like to split those calories up into a few meals because it helps them to better manage their hunger. You can go with whatever method you would like as long as you are able to stay within the calorie allotment that you are given.

When choosing your meals, make sure that you are going with healthier options. You can pick a big piece of cake to cover your 500 calories if you'd like, but you probably won't feel full or satisfied afterwards. When you feel hungry, a short time later you will likely regret your decision to indulge. Making wise decisions while fasting puts yourself in a better position to manage your hunger.

You should choose one or two days during the week to fast; you will not want to do more than this during the week. In addition, make sure that you split the days up so that you do not have two fasting days back to back; this is key to preventing your body from panicking from a lack of food, putting you into starvation mode. The best way to choose when to fast is to pick two days during your week when you expect to be pretty busy and use those as your fasting days. When you keep busy with work, it will help keep your mind off food and hunger.

Moving on to the non-fasting days, these are going to be your regular days, when you will not have to fast or worry about your calories as much. However, you should still eat healthily and not to go crazy with the number of calories that you consume when you're on your non-fasting days. Otherwise, you will minimize the benefits that you are getting from those fasting days.

Ultimately, you want to make sure that you are eating normally on the non-fasting days. Your focus should be on eating healthy foods such as vegetables, fruits, whole grains, nuts, seeds, and lean, white meats, since these will provide you with the essential minerals and nutrients. However, outside of your fasting days, you will not need to worry about counting the calories as much.

Chapter 5: Fasting Day Recipes

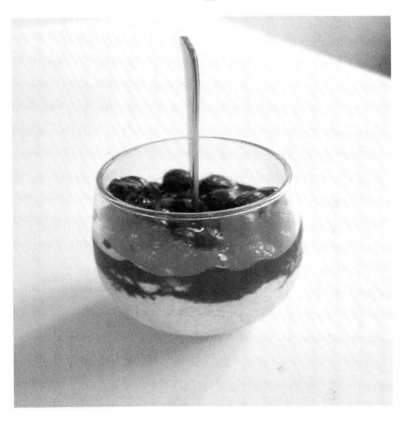

Blueberry Compote and Yogurt

This is a great recipe that you are going to want to make all the time on your fasting days. It only takes a few minutes to make and is perfect for when you're trying to get out of the door in the morning.

What's in it

- Bran (1 tsp.)
- Fat-free yogurt (3 Tbsp.)
- Blueberries (50 pcs.)

How's it done

1. Take out a bowl and place the blueberries inside.
2. Place the bowl in the microwave and heat on a high setting for about 45 seconds so that the blueberries will start to burst.
3. Take the bowl out of the microwave and let it cool down a bit.
4. When the blueberries are cooked, top with the bran and the yogurt before serving.

Notes:

You can also choose to make this with other berries and fruits (such as raspberries, blackberries, bananas, etc.) if you would like, though it may change the calorie count slightly.

Nutrition:

Calories: 75

Carbs: 11 g

Fat: 5 g

Protein: 1 g

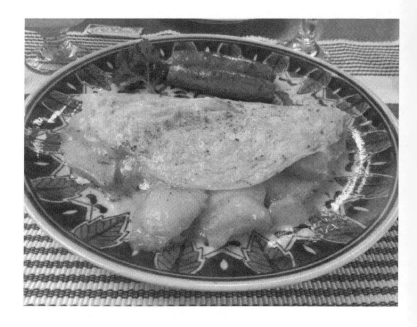

Swiss and Pear Omelet

This is a delicious omelet that is sure to fill you up no matter what time of day it is. You can have it as a hot breakfast or save it for the end of the day as a quick snack.

What's in it
- Shredded Swiss cheese (1.5 oz.)
- Almond milk (1.5 Tbsp.)
- Eggs (3 pcs.)
- Salt (0.25 tsp.)
- Chopped pear (0.25 pc.)

- Diced shallot (1 pc.)
- Olive oil (1 Tbsp.)

How's it done

1. Heat up a skillet. While it's heating up, chop up a pear into thin slices.
2. When the skillet is warm, add the salt, chopped pear, and shallot and cook for 5 minutes.
3. While that is cooking, take out a bowl and whisk together the almond milk and eggs. Pour this on top of the chopped pear to cook.
4. Once you see that the edges are turning white and the bottom has started to cook, flip your omelet over.
5. Add the cheese to the middle and fold the omelet in half. Cook a bit longer to melt the cheese.

Notes:

This omelet tastes great with other fruits as well if you would like to mix it up.

Nutrition:

Calories: 121

Carbs: 8 g

Fat: 12 g

Protein: 14 g

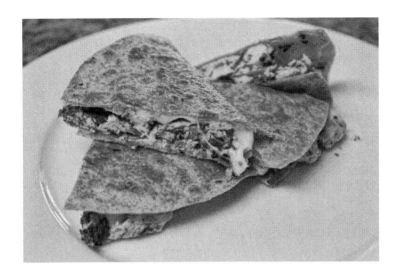

Breakfast Quesadillas

These quesadillas are simple and can be completed in a few minutes, making them perfect for all of your fasting days.

What's in it

- Chopped green onion (1 pc.)
- Egg (1 pc.)
- Tortilla (1 pc.)
- Salt
- Chili powder
- Water (0.5 Tbsp.)
- Chunky salsa (0.5 Tbsp.)

- Refried beans (0.5 Tbsp.)
- Cheddar cheese (2 Tbsp.)

How's it done

1. Start by whisking the water and the egg together with the chili powder.
2. Place a skillet over the stove and heat it up. Cook the green onion until it is tender and then reduce the heat to a medium setting.
3. Pour your egg mixture into this and then stir around until it is the desired consistency. Turn the heat off and cover this up to keep it warm.
4. On a clean counter, spread the tortilla out and add the salsa and beans. Add the egg on top of this and then top it all with cheese.
5. Wipe the skillet clean and place on a low flame. Heat this through, then add the quesadilla, and cook for a few minutes on each side.
6. Move the dish to a plate and then keep it warm before serving.

Notes:

Make a few servings of this at a time and then freeze the leftovers to use later on. This can make meal preparation even easier.

Nutrition:

Calories: 190

Carbs: 25 g

Fat: 11 g

Protein: 8 g

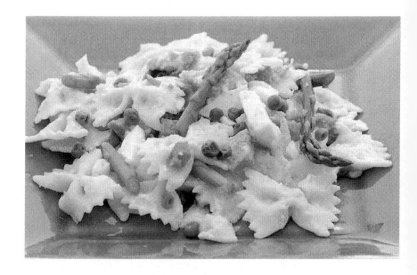

Ham and Asparagus Casserole

Nothing tastes better than a nice casserole in the morning. This one makes four servings so you can choose to eat it with your family or save it for later.

What's in it

- Cheddar cheese (0.5 c.)
- Cooked ham (0.5 c.)
- Flour (0.5 c.)
- Nonfat milk (1 c.)
- Chopped asparagus (2 pcs.)
- Eggs (4 pcs.)
- Chopped red bell pepper (1 pc.)

- Chopped onion (1 pc.)
- Pepper
- Salt
- Tarragon (0.25 tsp.)
- Parmesan (2 Tbsp.)

How's it done

1. Allow the oven to heat up to 425 degrees. Grease up a baking dish with cooking spray. Spread out the ham on the bottom and then follow with the bell pepper, onion, and asparagus.
2. Take out a bowl and whisk together the salt, pepper, dried tarragon, milk, flour, Parmesan cheese, and eggs.
3. When the egg mixture is mixed, pour it over the other ingredients inside your baking dish. Add the baking dish to the oven and let it bake.
4. After 10 minutes, the casserole should be set and you can take it out of the oven. Add the cheddar cheese and then bake two more minutes so the cheese can melt.
5. Allow it to stand on the cooling rack for a few minutes before serving.

Notes:

This casserole tastes great either warm or cold, so consider taking it to work on your fasting days.

Nutrition:

Calories: 190

Carbs: 5 g

Fat: 11 g

Protein: 12 g

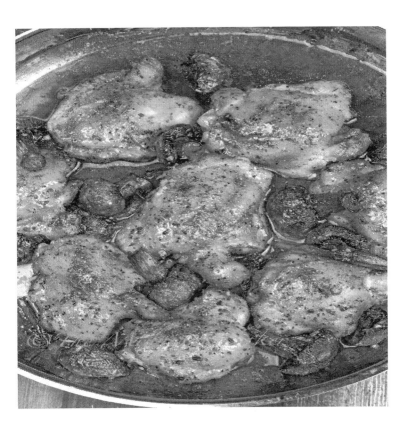

Italian Chicken

There is nothing easier than throwing a nice chicken dinner together. The chicken will provide you with enough protein to keep you full on your fasting days.

What's in it
- Cooking spray
- Salt
- Pepper

- Italian seasoning (0.5 tsp.)
- Balsamic vinegar(1 Tbsp.)
- Feta cheese (2 Tbsp.)
- Sliced Roma tomato (1 pc.)
- Chicken breasts (2 pcs.)

How's it done

1. Turn on the oven to a broil setting. Take out your broiler pan and spray it with some cooking spray.
2. Rinse the chicken off and then blot dry with some paper towels. Season the chicken with the pepper, salt, and Italian seasoning.
3. Lay the chicken onto your prepared broiler pan and then broil for 5 minutes on each side until the chicken reaches 165 degrees.
4. Place two tomato slices on each chicken breast and add the cheese to the top. Spoon the balsamic vinegar over it all.
5. Place this back into the oven and let it broil for another 3 minutes until the cheese is pale brown. Move to a serving dish and serve.

Notes:

You can try adding a different type of cheese like Cheddar or Pepper Jac to this to give a different flavoring to the whole dish.

Nutrition:

Calories: 220

Carbs: 11 g

Fat: 12 g

Protein: 23 g

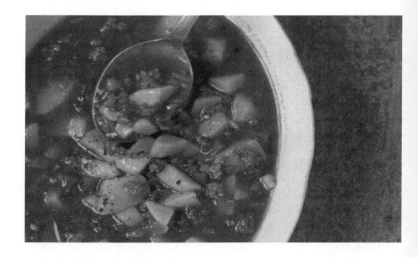

Potato and Beef Soup

Nothing tastes better and fills you up more than some nice, hot soup on a cold day. Add this dish to your meal plan for fasting days. Feel free to make a large batch and store portions in the freezer for an easy meal later.

What's in it
- Cooking spray
- Cumin (0.5 tsp.)
- Chopped cilantro (2 tbsp.)
- Red or Yukon Gold potatoes (1.5 c.)
- Water (1.5 c.)
- Diced tomatoes (2 c.)

- Diced onion (1 pc.)
- Beef sirloin steak (0.5 lb.)

How's it done

1. Rinse off the beef steak and blot it dry. Slice into smaller cubes and set aside.
2. Coat the inside of a heavy stew pot with some cooking spray and then set it on the stove to get hot.
3. Add in the prepared beef to the stew pot and cook until the pieces are browned all over which will take about five minutes. Stir in the onion and let it cook until it is tender.
4. Stir in the water, cumin, and tomatoes. Mix this well and bring it to a boil. When this is boiling, reduce the temperatore to medium and then cover and simmer for about 20 minutes.
5. Uncover the pot and then stir in the cubed potatoes. Cover this and let it simmer for a bit longer until both the beef and the potatoes are tender, which will take another 10 minutes.
6. At this time, turn the heat off and let it stand, with the cover on, for about 5 minutes.

7. Ladle this into some soup bowls and then serve.

Notes:

Double this recipe and then freeze it to use on another day when you are busy. You can also add some more vegetables, like peas and carrots to make this a healthier option to go with for just a few more calories.

Nutrition:

Calories: 200

Carbs: 10 g

Fat: 11 g

Protein: 12 g

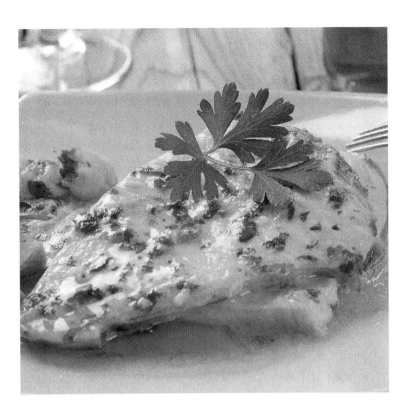

Lemon Flounder

Consider adding more fish to your diet even on your fasting days. This one is going to be so satisfying and will help you get all the nutrition that you need to keep you healthy and happy.

cookie

What's in it

- Snow peas, chopped (0.25 c.)

- Baby corn (0.25 c.)
- Diced carrots (0.25 c.)
- Baby peas (0.25 c.)
- Chicken broth (0.75 c.)
- Red onion, sliced (0.5)
- Halved flounder fillet (0.5 lb.)
- Drill, dried (0.25 tsp.)
- Lemon pepper seasoning (1 tsp.)
- Cornstarch (1 Tbsp.)

How's it done

1. To get started with this recipe, take out a pan and heat it up to a high heat on the stove. Pour on the chicken broth before adding the lemon pepper seasoning, dill, and sliced onion.
2. Cover and let this simmer for another 3 minutes until the onion is tender.
3. Uncover the pan and then stir in the snow peas, corn, diced carrots, and baby peas. Add the flounder to the top of the ingredients and simmer for another 5 minutes so that the fish can cook all the way through.
4. Move the fish to a bowl using a slotted spoon and then cover to keep the fish warm.

5. Take a bit of the broth out of the soup and add to the bowl. Stir in the cornstarch before adding this back to the pan. Stir it well and bring to a boil.
6. Pour the broth and vegetables on top of the fish and then serve.

Notes:

You can add a nice side salad with some homemade dressing if you still need to get a few calories to get to your 500 or 600 calories for the day.

Nutrition:

Calories: 190

Carbs: 2 g

Fat: 10 g

Protein: 14 g

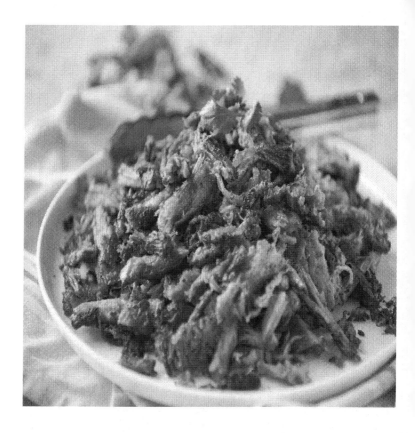

Pork Carnitas

These pork carnitas are quick and easy to make. You can always save yourself time by making extra pork and freezing it - you'll thank yourself later when you feel tired from a busy day and the only thing you'll have to do is reheat your leftovers.

What's in it

- Pepper
- Salt (0.25 tsp.)
- Dark molasses (0.5 Tbsp.)
- Orange juice (0.5 Tbsp.)
- Brown sugar (1 Tbsp.)
- Minced garlic clove (1 pc.)
- Pork tenderloin (0.5 lb.)

How's it done

1. Rinse off the pork tenderloin and blot it down with some paper towels. Slice thinly and then set it aside.
2. Place a skillet on a flame and then heat it through. Once it is hot, add the pork tenderloin. Cook these for about 4 minutes until the pork is tender and cook it through.
3. Drain out the oil before stirring in the pepper, salt, molasses, orange juice, and brown sugar.
4. Stir this around and simmer until your sauce is thick. Turn off the heat and let it stand for a few minutes to thicken before serving.

Notes:

You can add a little bit more garlic to the mix if you feel that you need some more flavor to the meal. Add the pork to a few tortillas or to some lettuce leaves to complete the meal.

Nutrition:

Calories: 180

Carbs:: 2 g

Fat: 9 g

Protein: 14 g

Chapter 6: Nonfasting Day Breakfasts

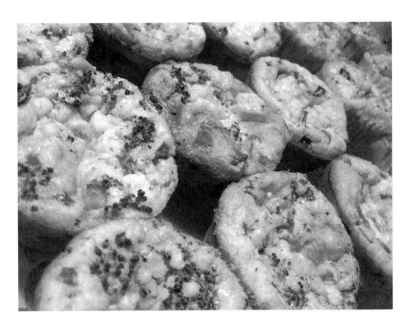

Mini Quiche's

Quiches are easy to make, and they are perfect if you're on the go. Perfect for breakfast or a mid-day snack, these quiches have all the protein you need to stay satisfied all day long.

What's in it

- Olive oil (2 tsp.)
- Pepper (0.25 tsp.)
- Salt (0.5 tsp.)
- Rosemary (1 Tbsp.)
- Parmesan cheese (0.75 c.)
- Egg whites (6 pcs.)
- Eggs (5 pcs.)
- Cooking spray
- Baby spinach (3 oz.)
- Mushrooms (6 oz.)
- Minced garlic cloves (1 pc.)
- Chopped red onion (0.5 pc.)

How's it done

1. Turn on the oven and allow it to heat up to 350 degrees. Coat some muffin tins with cooking spray and add some liners into each one.

2. In a bowl, whisk together the pepper, salt, rosemary, Parmesan cheese, egg whites, and eggs to make them fluffy.

3. Take out a skillet and heat up the olive oil inside. Add the garlic and onion until they are fragrant. Now add in the mushrooms and then cook for another 5 minutes.

4. Take the pan off the heat and let it cool down a little bit. Place some of this mixture into each of the prepared muffin cups and add some spinach on the top.
5. Slowly pour the egg mixture into each cup and fill to the rim. Add these to the oven and let them bake.
6. After 25 minutes, take them out of the oven and allow them to cool down before serving.

Notes:

You will find that by using some paper muffin liners to make the quiche, you can save time on clean up.

Nutrition (1 mini quiche):

Calories: 83

Carbs: 2 g

Fat: 5 g

Protein: 8 g

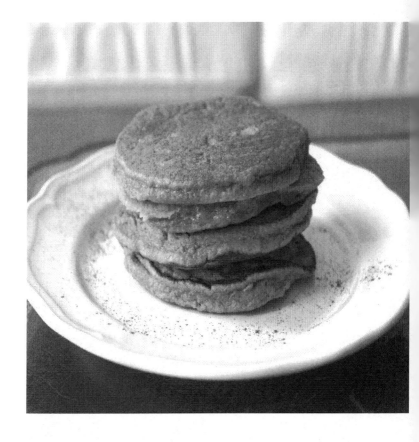

Sweet Potato Pancakes

These pancakes pack 18 grams of protein in each serving and offer plenty of vitamins to keep you healthy and strong. This quick and easy meal is a fantastic, balanced breakfast to start your day off great.

What's in it

- Maple syrup (1.5 Tbsp.)
- Nutmeg (0.25 tsp.)
- Cinnamon (1 tsp.)
- Egg whites (4 pcs.)
- Eggs (5 pcs.)
- Oats (1.5 c.)
- Cottage cheese (1.5 c.)
- Sweet potatoes (2 pcs.)

How's it done

1. Allow the oven some time to heat up to 400 degrees. Take your potatoes and prick them a few times with a fork. Add them to a baking sheet and let them cook for a bit.
2. After 50 minutes, take the potatoes out of the oven and carefully slit them lengthwise. Allow these to cool a bit before scooping the flesh of the potatoes into the blender.
3. Add the syrup, nutmeg, cinnamon, egg whites, eggs, oats, and cottage cheese into the blender. Blend this until it is smooth.
4. Now, take out a big skillet and prepare it with some cooking spray. When this is hot, after two minutes, scoop some of the batter onto the

skillet and cook so that the pancakes become golden brown, which will take about 4 minutes on each side.

5. Repeat with the rest of the batter and then serve warm.

Notes:

You can make this recipe a few times and then store in the freezer for up to 3 months. This makes it easier for you to just defrost them the night before and have them ready for those busy days.

Nutrition:

Calories: 238

Carbs: 28 g

Fat: 6 g

Protein: 18 g

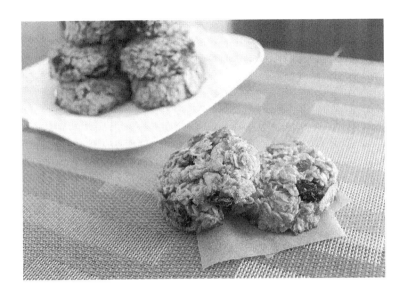

Cherry and Almond Breakfast Cookies

Who would have thought that cookies can make a healthy breakfast? These small cookies are full of fruit, nuts, and whole grains which provide an excellent source of nutrition in the morning. These are also great to take with you and eat on the go.

What's in it

- Baking soda (1 tsp.)
- Whole-wheat flour (2.25 c.)
- Rolled oats (0.5 c.)
- Cooking spray
- Sliced raw almonds (1 c.)

- Chopped tart cherries, dried (1 c.)
- Vanilla (1 tsp.)
- Eggs (2 pcs.)
- Maple syrup (0.5 c.)
- Brown sugar (0.5 c.)
- Plain Greek yogurt (0.5 c.)
- Applesauce (0.5 c.)
- Salt (0.25 tsp.)

How's it done

1. Allow the oven to heat up to 350 degrees. Take a few baking sheets and line with some parchment paper.
2. Take out a bowl and combine the salt, baking soda, flour, and oats.
3. In a second bowl, whisk together the Greek yogurt and applesauce. When those are mixed, add the maple syrup and brown sugar until the mixture is smooth. Add the vanilla and the eggs and mix to smooth the mixture together.
4. Slowly fold the dry ingredients into the wet ones and stir to combine. Now, add the almonds and cherries, making sure that they are well distributed in the batter.

5. Add 2 tablespoons of batter onto a baking sheet to make each cookie and then flatten them down a little bit. Place in the oven to bake.
6. After 15 minutes, you can take the cookies out and let them cool before serving or storing.

Notes:

You will find that these tart cherries are a great source of a lot of nutrients that the body needs. Eating a few of these each day will help you to get going and feel great, even while cheating a little bit.

Nutrition:

Calories: 214

Carbs: 36 g

Fat: 6 g

Protein: 6 g

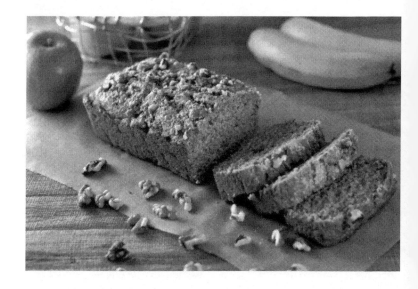

Apple Walnut Loaf

This is going to remind you of all the delicious food that you enjoyed at grandma's house when you were younger. Made with healthy ingredients, you can enjoy this tasty treat without worrying that you might consume too many calories.

What's in it

- Applesauce (0.5 c.)
- Cinnamon (0.5 tsp.)
- Salt (0.5 tsp.)
- Baking soda (1 tsp.)
- All-purpose flour (1 c.)

- Whole-wheat flour (1 c.)
- Cooking spray
- Chopped walnuts (0.5 c.)
- Chopped Rome apple (1 pc.)
- Unsweetened almond milk (0.5 c.)
- Egg (1 pc.)
- Honey (0.5 c.)

How's it done

1. Allow the oven to heat up to 325 degrees. Prepare a loaf pan with some cooking spray.
2. Take out a medium bowl and sift together the all-purpose and whole-wheat flours with the cinnamon, salt, and baking soda.
3. In another bowl, combine the honey and applesauce and stir it together until it is combined. Add the almond milk and egg and stir well.
4. Fold the dry ingredients into this, but be careful about overmixing. Fold in the walnuts and the apples in as well, making sure to distribute them throughout the batter.

5. Pour this batter into a loaf pan and spread it out evenly. Add this to the oven and allow to bake for almost an hour.

6. After 55 minutes, you can take the pan out of the oven and cool for 5 minutes and slice it up.

Notes:

You can keep this in a plastic container at room temperature for up to 5 days or freeze for a few days as well to eat later.

Nutrition:

Calories: 206

Carbs: 45 g

Fat: 2 g

Protein: 5 g

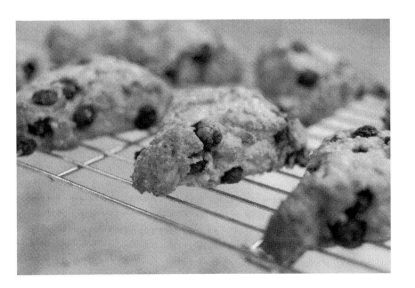

Blueberry Scones

It is hard to give up those sweet treats when you are on a diet. With these scones, you'll have the perfect excuse to satisfy your sweet tooth without feeling guilty. These scones are packed full of nutritious ingredients like Greek yogurt, whole-grains, and blueberries.

What's in it

- Salt (0.5 tsp.)
- Baking powder (4 tsp.)
- Whole-wheat flour (0.75 c.)
- Flour (1.25 c.)
- Cooking spray

- Wild blueberries (1 c.)
- Vanilla (1 tsp.)
- Milk (0.5 c.)
- Greek yogurt (1 c.)
- Canola oil (3 Tbsp.)
- Egg (1 pc.)
- Sugar (0.5 c.)
- Baking soda (0.25)

How's it done

1. Allow the oven to heat up to 400 degrees. Take out two baking sheets and cover with cooking spray.
2. In a bowl, sift together both the flours with the baking soda, salt, and baking powder.
3. In a second bowl, add the vanilla, milk, yogurt, oil, egg, and sugar. Fold the dry ingredients in with the wet ingredients until they are combined.
4. Fold in the blueberries and the drop some of the batter onto the baking sheets. Place the baking pans into the oven.
5. After 15 minutes, take the scones out of the oven and let them cool down before serving.

Notes:

When blueberries are not in season, it is fine to go with frozen ones. The wild blueberries are good to add into the scones because they have plenty of nutrients and antioxidants that your body needs to get going in the morning.

Nutrition:

Calories: 160

Carbs: 26 g

Fat: 4 g

Protein: 5 g

Chapter 7: Nonfasting Day Lunches

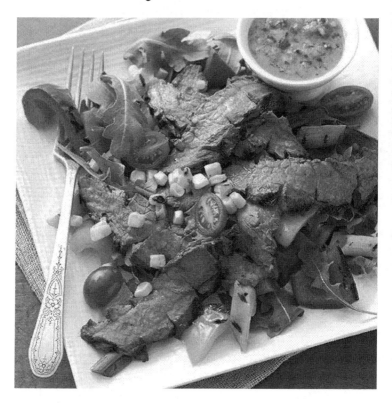

Grilled Steak Salad

There is nothing as satisfying to eat for lunch than this salad. With fresh greens to provide you with the right vitamins, minerals, and healthy protein to keep you strong, you'll be sure to enjoy this favorite again and again.

What's in it

- Cucumber, sliced (1 pc.)
- Halved cherry tomatoes (1 c.)
- Mixed greens (1 package)
- Flank steak (1 lb.)
- Soy sesame dressing
- Grated carrot (1 pc.)

How's it done

1. Take out a bowl and add in the steak with some of the dressing. Make sure that all your steak is covered with the dressing and then set aside for a minimum of 30 minutes to marinate.
2. After the steak has had some time to marinate, turn on the grill, and get it preheated. Place the steak on the grill and get rid of the extra marinade.
3. Let the steak grill until it reaches 145 degrees, which will take about 5 minutes on each side. Move the steak to a plate and allow the steak to rest for a bit before slicing.
4. Place some of the greens on four different plates and top with the carrots, cucumbers, and tomatoes. Layer the steak across the bowl.

Drizzle with some of the dressing and then serve.

Notes:

You can make your own mixed greens if you like. You can add in any combination of greens, such as arugula, butter lettuce, red lead lettuce, radicchio, and spinach.

Nutrition:

Calories: 433

Carbs: 10 g

Fat: 35 g

Protein: 24 g

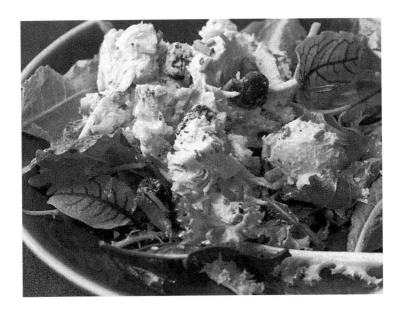

Turkey Walnut Salad

If you have any extra turkey leftover from another meal, especially around the holidays, this is a fantastic recipe for you to try. It's easy to put together and will help you feel satisfied when fasting.

What's in it

- Chopped walnuts (0.25 c.)
- Chopped celery (1 pc.)
- Chopped yellow onion (0.5 pc.)
- Minced turkey (8 oz.)
- Pepper

- Salt
- Parsley (2 tsp.)
- Lemon juice (1 tsp.)
- Dijon mustard (1 Tbsp.)
- Greek yogurt (2 Tbsp.)
- Mayo (2 Tbsp.)
- Dried cranberries (3 Tbsp.)

How's it done

1. Take out a bowl and combine the cranberries, walnuts, celery, onion, and turkey.
2. In another bowl, combine the pepper, salt, parsley, lemon juice, mustard, Greek yogurt, and mayo.
3. Top this second bowl on top of the turkey mixture and stir it well before serving.

Notes:

If you are worried about how much mayo is inside the bowl, and the extra calories it contains, you can substitute with some Greek yogurt.

Nutrition:

Calories: 175

Carbs: 8 g

Fat: 8 g

Protein: 17 g

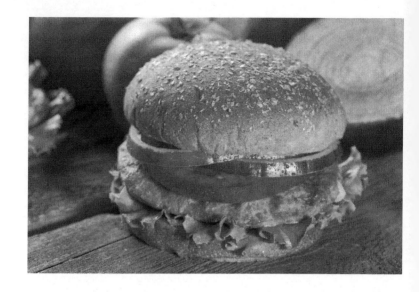

Turkey Burgers

Turkey Burgers hit all the right notes for a traditionally satisfying meal. High in protein, quick, and easy, this is sure to be a favorite for lunch or dinner. The feta and the spinach help bind the burgers together and will add a little more flavor to the dish. Enjoy with some yogurt as a sauce to give your burger a whole new layer of taste.

What's in it
- Cooking spray
- Pepper (0.25 tsp.
- Dried oregano (1 tsp.)
- Minced garlic clove (1 pc.)

- Feta (0.25 c.)
- Chopped red onion (0.25)
- Spinach (6 oz.)
- Ground turkey (1 lb.)
- *Yogurt sauce*
- Minced garlic clove (0.5)
- Salt (0.25 tsp.)
- Dill (1 Tbsp.)
- Lemon juice (2 Tbsp.)
- Greek yogurt (1 c.)

How's it done

1. Start by making the burger patties. Take out a bowl and combine the pepper, oregano, garlic, feta, onion, spinach, and turkey.
2. Use your hands to form this mixture into four patties.
3. Add some cooking spray to the grill and then add the burger patties onto it. Cook these on a high temperature until they reach 165 degrees which takes about five minutes on each side.
4. When the burgers are done, take them off the grill and set aside to cool.

5. Now, it's time to make the yogurt sauce. Take out a bowl and combine the salt, dill, lemon juice, Greek yogurt, and garlic. Stir the ingredients until they are combined.
6. When you are ready to serve, top some of this yogurt sauce on top of each burger.

Notes:

You can choose to place your burger on a whole grain bun with some of your favorite toppings such as tomato and lettuce.

Nutrition:

Calories: 248

Carbs: 6 g

Fat: 12 g

Protein: 30 g

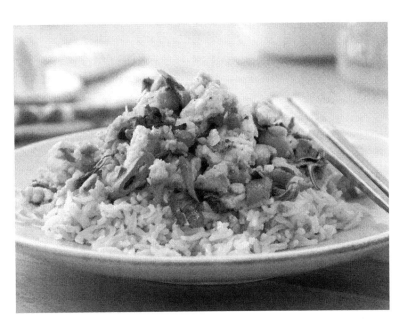

Thai Chicken Stir Fry

Stir-fries are one of the best things that you can make when you need to feed the whole family that is fresh, easy, and quick. They also allow you to introduce some different flavors to the meal to keep things new and interesting.

What's in it
- Brown rice (1 c.)
- Water (3 c.)
- Thai marinade (0.33 c.)
- Chicken breast, sliced (1.25 lbs.)

- Sliced red bell pepper (1 pc.)
- Sliced white mushrooms (8 oz.)
- Sliced broccoli (0.5 head)
- Canola oil (1 Tbsp.)

How's it done

1. Take out a big bowl and add the chicken strips with your marinade. Toss around to coat, then cover the bowl, and let it marinate for at least 30 minutes or overnight.
2. Now, boil some water in a medium pot. Add the brown rice and lower the heat a little bit to medium. Cover and let the rice simmer for 40 minutes so that it becomes tender.
3. After about 40 minutes, drain out the extra water and then move the rice over to a bowl to let it cool.
4. Take out a skillet and heat up the oil until it starts to shimmer. Add the chicken, without the leftover marinade, and cook so that it browns on all sides.
5. Now, add the bell pepper, mushrooms, and broccoli. Let these cook until they start to soften, which will take about 8 minutes.

6. Add some of the reserved marinade and cook another minute before serving.

Notes:

If you have a rice cooker, you can choose to use that to cook your rice. This recipe also works to help with some other grains as well, such as quinoa and farro.

Nutrition:

Calories: 357

Carbs: 46 g

Fat: 3 g

Protein: 24 g

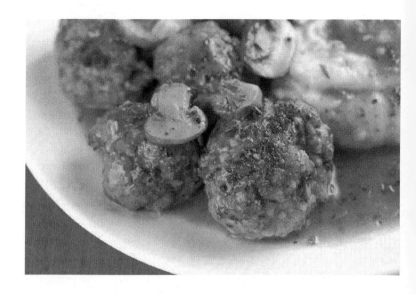

Beef Mushroom Meatballs

These mushroom meatballs are perfect for your fasting days. Their compact size means they can be eaten as a snack, added to a salad, or served as the main dish.

What's in it

- Minced garlic cloves (2 pc.)
- Parsley, chopped (0.5 c.)
- Breadcrumbs (0.75 c.)
- Ground beef (1 lb.)
- Chopped Portobello mushrooms (1 container)
- Safflower oil (1 Tbsp.)

- Pepper (0.25 tsp.)
- Salt (0.25 tsp.)
- Beaten egg (1 pc.)

How's it done

1. To start this recipe, take a skillet out and heat up some oil until it is shimmering. Add the chopped mushrooms, cook them for 5 minutes to soften them up, and then remove the mushrooms from the heat so they can cool down.

2. Turn on the oven and allow it to heat up to 350 degrees. Take out a bowl and combine the pepper, salt, egg, garlic, parsley, breadcrumbs, beef, and mushrooms. Mix these together with your hands.

3. Form this mixture into balls and then place into muffin cups. Place in the oven and let them bake.

4. After 25 minutes, take the meatballs out of the oven and let them cool before serving or storing.

Notes:

When you are ready to mix the ground beef together with the mushrooms, you will find that a ratio of 1 to 1 is the best to get good flavor.

Nutrition:

Calories: 232

Carbs: 12 g

Fat: 12 g

Protein: 19 g

Chapter 8: Nonfasting Day Dinners

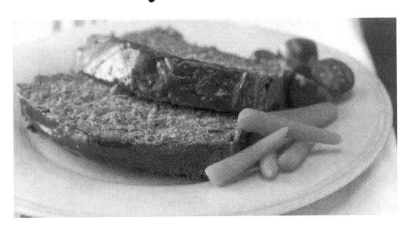

Beef and Lentil Meatloaf

Ground beef blends go well with legumes and vegetable to make this a healthy yummy dish. Besides, who doesn't love having a meatloaf for supper!?

What's in it

- Lentils (1 can)
- Minced garlic clove (1 pc.)
- Chopped onion (0.5 pc.)
- Chopped mushrooms (1 container)

- Ground beef (1 lb.)
- Tomato sauce (0.75 c.)
- Pepper (0.25 tsp.)
- Salt (0.5 tsp.)
- Panko bread crumbs (1 c.)
- Beaten egg (1 pc.)
- Cilantro (0.5 c.)

How's it done

1. Allow the oven to heat up to 350 degrees. Take out a loaf pan and spray it with some cooking spray.
2. Take out a bowl and mix the pepper, salt, panko, egg, cilantro, lentils, garlic, onions, mushrooms, and beef together.
3. Place the meat mixture into a loaf pan and get the top to be even. Pour the tomato sauce over the top. Add the pan to the oven.
4. Bake this for about an hour until the meatloaf is cooked all the way through. Let it cool down and slice into eight portions for serving.

Notes:

Panko is basically Japanese for breadcrumbs. If you have any extra bread or other bread crumbs around the house, it is fine to use those as well.

Nutrition:

Calories: 210

Carbs: 18 g

Fat: 7 g

Protein: 19 g

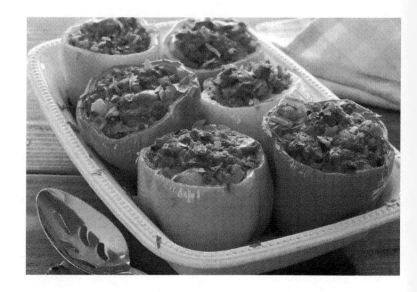

Stuffed Pepper

Stuffed peppers are a homemade classic that you will want to make over and over again. This version includes more whole grains, legumes, and veggies to give you more nutrients. You can add other ingredients to the stuffing to make something new for dinner every night.

What's in it
- Chickpeas (1 c.)
- Ground beef (1 lb.)
- Cooking spray
- Farro (1 c.)

- Water (3 c.)
- Bell peppers, any color (8 pcs.)
- Pepper (0.25 tsp.)
- Salt (0.5 tsp.)
- Lemon juice (1 Tbsp.)
- Olive oil (3 Tbsp.)
- Feta cheese (0.33 c.)
- Chopped yellow onion (0.5)
- Chopped parsley (1 bunch)
- Cherry tomatoes (1 c.)

How's it done

1. Take out a pot and bring two cups of water to a boil. Add the farro and let it to simmer until all the water is absorbed and your grain is tender, which takes 30 minutes.
2. After the farro is done cooking, drain off the excess liquid and allow it to cool down for a bit. Cover and let it set in the fridge for 30 minutes.
3. Turn on the oven and heat it up to 350 degrees. Prepare a baking dish with some cooking spray.
4. Take out a big bowl and combine the onion, parsley, tomatoes, chickpeas, and beef. Then add the feta cheese and the chilled farro.

5. In a small bowl, whisk together the black pepper, salt, lemon juice, and olive oil. Pour this mixture in with your beef mixture and stir to combine.
6. Take out your peppers and slice the tops off. Remove all the membranes and the seeds from the peppers and then spoon in the beef mixture.
7. Add the peppers to a baking dish, leaving a little bit of room between them. Cover this dish with some foil and then place into the oven to bake.
8. After 50 minutes, take the foil from the baking dish and let these bake for a little bit longer. After 20 more minutes, you can take them out and serve.

Notes:

You are able to store the cooled down peppers inside a dish for up to 2 months and let them thaw overnight. You can reheat a pepper in the microwave for a few minutes and then serve.

Nutrition:

Calories: 320

Carbs: 30 g

Fat: 14 g

Protein: 19 g

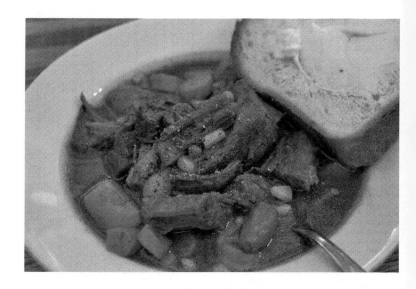

Beef Stew

On cold nights, nothing tastes better than some beef stew on the stove. You can also consider adding green beans or peppers to add more flavor to the dish.

What's in it

- Beef stew meat (1.5 lb.)
- Sweet potatoes (1.25 lbs.)
- Chickpeas (1 can)
- Pepper (0.25 tsp.)
- Salt (0.25 tsp.)
- Paprika (1 tsp.)

- Dried thyme (1 tsp.)
- Worcestershire sauce (1 Tbsp.)
- Tomato paste (2 Tbsp.)
- Beef broth (2.5 c.)
- Bay leaves (3 pcs.)
- Minced garlic cloves (2 pcs.)
- Diced celery stalk (1 pc.)
- Diced yellow onion (1 pc.)
- Peas (1 c.)
- Baby carrots (1 c.)

How's it done

1. Take out your slow cooker and add the bay leaves, garlic, celery, onion, peas, carrots, sweet potatoes, chickpeas, and meat inside.
2. In a bowl, whisk together the pepper, salt, paprika, thyme, Worcestershire sauce, tomato paste, and beef broth. Pour this mixture into the slow cooker.
3. Cover up the slow cooker and then cook on a high setting for about 6 hours and serve.

Notes:

This beef stew is considered almost like a soup because it is a little thinner. If you would like to make it thicker, you can add in some of the liquid from the slow cooker with some flour and then stir back into the stew. Cook for another 30 minutes before serving.

Nutrition:

Calories: 518

Carbs: 59 g

Fat: 10 g

Protein: 49 g

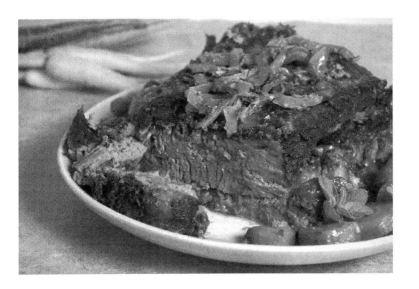

Slow Cooker Brisket

Slow cooker meals are the best for those busy days. Just throw the meat in the slow cooker in the morning and come home to a delicious home cooked meal.

What's in it

- Lager beer (1 bottle)
- Beef brisket (3 lb.)
- Pepper (0.25 tsp.)
- Salt (0.5 tsp.)
- Cumin (0.5 tsp.)
- Smoked paprika (0.5 tsp.)

- Instant coffee crystals (1 tsp.)
- Brown sugar (1 Tbsp.)

How's it done

1. Take out a bowl and combine the pepper, salt, cumin, paprika, coffee crystals, and brown sugar.
2. Using your hands, you can rub this mixture all over the brisket. Set up the slow cooker to a high setting before adding the brisket inside.
3. Pour the beer all over the brisket and then place the lid on top of the slow cooker.
4. Cover the slow cooker and cook it on high for about 6 hours. When the brisket is done, allow it to cool for about 10 minutes. Then slice or shred up the meat before serving.

Notes:

You can serve the brisket with any kind of side that you would like. Carrots, potatoes, sweet potatoes, or other vegetables can be nice. If you have a lot of leftovers, consider serving it for a baked potato, on a salad, or for tacos.

Nutrition:

Calories: 459

Carbs: 3 g

Fat: 13 g

Protein: 74 g

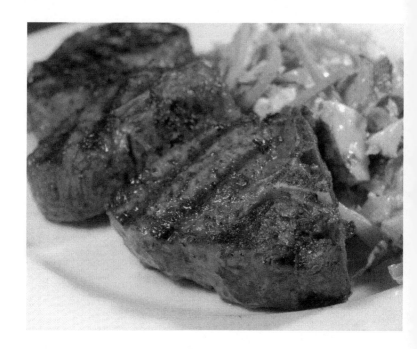

Lamb Chops

Lamb is a great source of protein to help keep your muscles strong. Add some vegetables to the mix, and you are sure to have a meal that you will want to try again and again.

What's in it

- Pepper (0.25 tsp.)
- Salt (0.25 tsp.)
- Dry white wine (2 Tbsp.)
- Greek yogurt (1 c.)
- Minced garlic cloves (4 pcs.)

- Mint leaves (0.75 c.)
- Lamb chops (8 pcs.)
- Cooking spray

How's it done

1. In a bowl, mix together some pepper, salt, all of the wine, half a cup of yogurt, three garlic cloves, and half a cup of mint.

2. Add the lamb to this and toss around to coat. Place this bowl in the fridge to marinate for about an hour.

3. Turn on your grill or prepare a grill pan with some cooking spray and place it over medium-high heat.

4. While your lamb is marinating, you can make the yogurt sauce. In a bowl, whisk together the pepper, salt, and the rest of the yogurt, garlic, and mint.

5. Take the lamb out of the marinade and place it onto the grill. Cook for about 12 minutes until the inside of the lamb reaches around 145 degrees.

6. When you are ready to serve, place two chops on a plate and have 2 tablespoons of yogurt sauce on the side to enjoy later.

Notes:

You can store any of the leftovers for about a week. This can make it an easy lunch when you are too busy to make something.

Nutrition:

Calories: 300

Carbs: 3 g

Fat: 4 g

Protein: 46 g

Chapter 9: Healthy Snacks to Help You Out

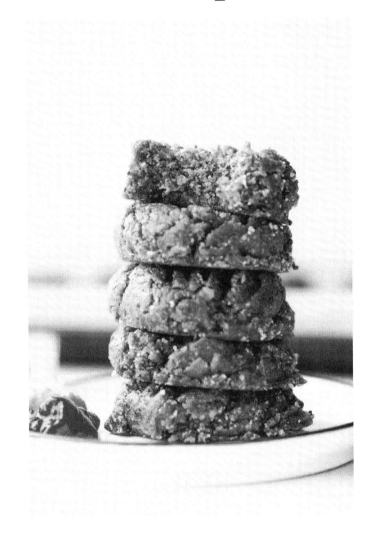

Peanut Butter Energy Cookies

For those times you find yourself craving something sweet, these cookies make the perfect healthy snack. These tasty treats are a healthy way to curb cravings while giving you a much-needed boost of energy.

What's in it

- Peanut butter, creamy (0.5 c.)
- Salt (0.25 tsp.)
- Baking soda (1 tsp.)
- Cocoa powder (0.25 c.)
- Flour (1 c.)
- Chopped peanuts (0.5 c.)
- Rolled oats (2 c.)
- Vanilla (1 tsp.)
- Beaten eggs (2 pcs.)
- Brown sugar (0.5 c.)
- Milk (0.5 c.)
- Greek yogurt (0.25 c.)
- Mashed banana (1 c.)

How's it done

1. Take out a bowl and sift together the salt, baking soda, cocoa powder, and flour.
2. In another bowl, stir together the milk, Greek yogurt, banana, and peanut butter. Add the brown sugar and then stir to combine. Now, add the vanilla and the eggs and combine.
3. Add the flour to this peanut butter mixture and then the oats and peanuts and mix this with the dry ingredients until moist. Cover the bowl and place in the fridge for 30 minutes.
4. Allow the oven to heat up to 350 degrees. Take out two baking sheets and coat with some baking spray.
5. Drop some of the batter onto the baking sheets and then press them down a little bit. Place in the oven to bake.
6. After about 15 minutes, you can take the cookies out of the oven and allow them to cool down before serving.

Notes:

You can make a few batches so that you always have some cookies ready when you want to snack.

Nutrition:

Calories: 143

Carbs: 19 g

Fat: 1 g

Protein: 5 g

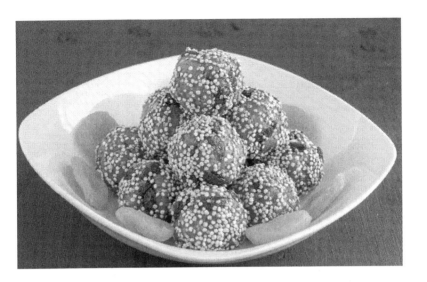

Orange and Apricot Bites

These bite-sized snacks are nutritious and delicious, and sure to satisfy your sweet tooth. These are also a great pick-me-up to help you through your day if you start to feel hungry.

What's in it

- Coconut (0.66 c.)
- Almond butter (0.5 c)
- Dried apricots (0.5 c.)
- Pitted dates (1.5 c.)
- Rolled oats (1 c.)
- Vanilla (1 tsp.)
- Orange juice (3 Tbsp.)

- Zest of an orange (1 Tbsp.)

How's it done

1. Allow the oven to heat up to 350 degrees. Line some parchment paper on a baking sheet. Place some oats on the baking sheet and toast them for a few minutes until they are slightly toasted.
2. While your oats are in the oven, take the food processor out and place the dates into the food processor and pulse to make smooth.
3. Add the vanilla, orange juice and zest, coconut, almond butter, apricots, and toasted oats to the food processor. Pulse so that the mixture becomes smooth. Move to a bowl.
4. Use your hands to make little balls out of the batter and place them into a resealable container. Allow these to set for at least 15 minutes and then serve.

Notes:

While the oats are gluten-free, it is important to realize that many brands will make these in a factory that may also work with gluten products. Look on the package to find out where your product is made.

Nutrition:

Calories: 117

Carbs: 17 g

Fat: 2 g

Protein: 3 g

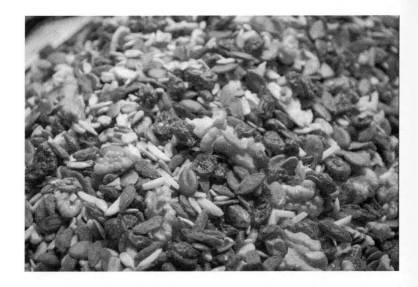

Trail Mix

Making your own trail mix puts you in full control. You can determine what ingredients go inside so you get the best tasting trail mix. Nibble on this snack when you start to feel hungry for a nutritious boost of energy.

What's in it

- Sunflower seeds (2 Tbsp.)
- Dark chocolate chips (3 Tbsp.)
- Dried tart cherries (3 Tbsp.)
- Dried apricots (10 pcs.)
- Raw almonds (0.5 c.)

How's it done

1. To get make your trail mix, take out a bowl and add the almonds, sunflower seeds, chocolate chips, cherries, and apricots.
2. Toss all these together and then add it to a resealable container. You are able to store it in there for up to a month.

Notes:

You can easily double or triple this recipe and then split it up into smaller portions so that it is ready to go whenever you are. You can also mix up the combination of dried fruit and nuts that you are using so that you get the taste that is right for you.

Nutrition:

Calories: 216

Carbs: 18 g

Fat: 15 g

Protein: 6 g

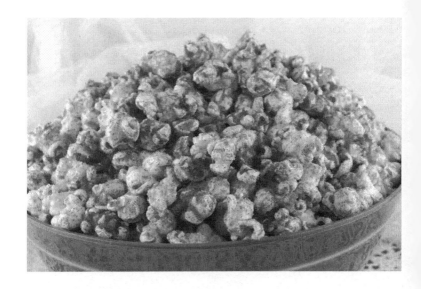

Cinnamon Cocoa Popcorn

There is nothing better to snack on than a little bit of popcorn. Adding chocolate and cinnamon to popcorn can make this healthy snack a little bit more fun. You can mix and match a variety of toppings to get the flavor that you like best.

What's in it
- Cinnamon (1 tsp.)
- Cocoa powder (1 Tbsp.)
- Cooking spray
- Popcorn kernels (0.5 c.)
- Coconut oil (3 Tbsp.)
- Salt (1 tsp.)

- Sugar (1 Tbsp.)

How's it done

1. Take a gallon pot out and heat up the three tablespoons of coconut oil. Add three popcorn kernels, and then when one of the kernels start to pop, you know that it is hot enough. Add in the rest of the kernels.
2. Cover the pot with its lid and shake it round to make sure that there isn't any burning. When the popcorn is popped, you can add the prepared popcorn to a mixing bowl.
3. Spray your popcorn with some cooking spray. Use your hands to toss the popcorn around to mix well.
4. Sprinkle with the salt, sugar, cinnamon, and cocoa powder. Make sure that the popcorn is coated properly before serving.

Notes:

Another option is to use an air popper to pop the kernels. You can then just toss the popcorn with some melted coconut oil in a bowl before adding in the flavors.

Nutrition:

Calories: 188

Carbs: 24 g

Fat: 12 g

Protein: 3 g

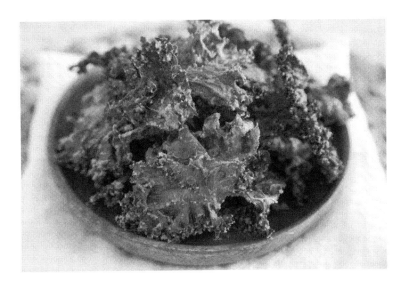

Kale Chips

Kale chips are all the rage for those who are looking for a healthier alternative to traditional potato chips. Buying kale chips in stores can be expensive, and you have no control over how it's made. This recipe allows you to make kale chips from the comfort of your home and save you money in the process.

What's in it

- Salt (1 tsp.)
- Lime juice (2 Tbsp.)
- Zest of a lime (1 pc.)
- Sriracha (1 tsp.)

- Olive oil (0.25 c.)
- Cooking spray
- Torn kale (1 bag)
- Pepper (0.5 tsp.)

How's it done

1. Turn on the oven and allow it to heat up to 400 degrees. Take out two baking pans and coat them with some cooking spray.
2. In a big bowl, whisk together the black pepper, salt, lime zest and juice, sriracha, and olive oil.
3. Take out the torn kale, add it to the bowl, and then toss around until the leaves have been coated with the dressing.
4. Pour the kale into single even layers on the baking sheet. Add to the oven and let them bake.
5. After about 10 minutes, the kale should be crisp. You can take them out of the oven and allow them to cool off.

Notes:

Buying the bags of kale that are already torn up can save you a ton of time. These are usually pretty reasonably priced at most grocery stores. If you want, you can also purchase a head of kale on your own and tear it up to make these chips.

Nutrition:

Calories: 102

Carbs: 5 g

Fat: 1 g

Protein: 1 g

Chapter 10: Seven Days to a Better You

Now that you have plenty of delicious recipes to keep you company on your intermittent fasting journey, it is time to learn about some of the ways you can ensure the process is as successful as possible. You are never going to be successful with this kind of fast if you do not take some time to plan things out. Never forget, when it comes to intermittent fasting, failing to plan is the same as planning to fail.

The good news is that with a little bit of planning, the entire process becomes far easier to manage and you will be able to deal with the challenges that come with going on a fast. Here we are going to provide you with a simple meal plan that you can follow when you are on the 5:2 fast. This will show you how to split up the days, but you can split them up, however, you would like. However, you end up splitting up your fasts, just make sure that you follow a plan that you can stick with regularly for the best results. What follows is a meal plan that you can follow when you are just getting started with intermittent fasting.

Day 1: Nonfasting Day

Breakfast: Mini Quiche's

Lunch: Grilled Steak Salad

Dinner: Beef and Lentil Meatloaf

Snack: Peanut Butter Energy Cookies

Nutrition for the day

Calories: 1200

Carbs: 49 g

Fat: 48 g

Protein: 56 g

Day 2: Fasting Day

Breakfast: Blueberry Compote and Yogurt

Lunch: Italian Chicken

Dinner: Lemony Flounder

Nutrition for the day

Calories: 485

Carbs: 24 g

Fat: 26 g

Protein: 38 g

Day 3: Nonfasting Day

Breakfast: Sweet Potato Pancakes

Lunch: Turkey Walnut Salad

Dinner: Stuffed Peppers

Snack: Orange and Apricot Bites

Nutrition for the day

Calories: 1100

Carbs: 83 g

Fat: 30 g

Protein: 57 g

Day 4: Nonfasting Day

Breakfast: Cherry and Almond Breakfast Cookies

Lunch: Turkey Burgers

Dinner: Beef Stew

Snack: Trail Mix

Nutrition for the day

Calories: 1196

Carbs: 119 g

Fat: 43 g

Protein: 91 g

Day 5: Fasting Day

Breakfast: Swiss and Pear Omelet

Lunch: Potato and Beef Soup

Dinner: Pork Carnitas

Nutrition for the day

Calories: 501

Carbs: 20 g

Fat: 32 g

Protein: 40 g

Day 6: Nonfasting Day

Breakfast: Apple Walnut Loaf

Lunch: Thai Chicken Stir Fry

Dinner: Slow Cooker Brisket

Snack: Cinnamon Cocoa Popcorn

Nutrition for the day

Calories: 1210

Carbs: 118 g

Fat: 30 g

Protein: 106 g

Day 7: Nonfasting Day

Breakfast: Blueberry Scones
Lunch: Beef Mushroom Meatballs
Dinner: Lamb Chops
Snack: Kale Chips

Nutrition for the day

Calories: 1300
Carbs: 51 g
Fat: 21 g
Protein: 73 g

Chapter 11: FAQs

Getting started with the intermittent fast is a new experience. We have been told for years that we need to eat a certain way, that we shouldn't miss out on meals because we are going to go into starvation mode, that we have to eat at certain times and so many times per day, or that we will have trouble with our metabolism and staying healthy. But with intermittent fasting, all of this is thrown out the window so that you can actually get your body to burn fat and lose weight with less effort.

Naturally, this means that you may have some questions when you are first getting started. This chapter is going to answer some of the questions you may have before getting started on the intermittent fast.

What is intermittent fasting?

Intermittent fasting is a practice that humans have been using for thousands of years as a means of achieving a higher consciousness or communing with a higher power. Recently, more and more people have been practicing intermittent fasting due to its effectiveness for weight loss and other health benefits. Proponents of this new type of targeted intermittent fasting enjoy it because it doesn't require sticking to a limiting meal plan or require counting calories to see serious results.

The reason that intermittent fasting is so useful comes from the basic fact that the body behaves quite differently when it's in a fed state compared to when it's in a fasting state. A fed state is any period where the body is currently absorbing nutrients from foods it's actively digesting. This state begins roughly 5 minutes after you have finished a meal and generally lasts for about 5 hours depending on the foods you consume. While your body is ccupied, it's also creating insulin which means it's more difficult for it to burn fat as easily as it otherwise might.

You can choose which type of intermittent fast you would like to go with. Keep in mind that you're also able to eat zero-calorie gum, water, diet soda, and coffee during your fasting periods to help keep the hunger pains at bay.

Will fasting make me store fat or put me into starvation mode?

No, this is a common misconception that a lot of people have about intermittent fasting. Your metabolism is actually quite hearty and as long as you get into a routine with the way you eat and stick with it, your metabolism will be able to adjust accordingly. There are many good reasons to fast including fat loss, insulin reduction, and so much more.

There are a few key points that you can look at to determine whether this is a good diet plan to go with. First, you are going to burn fat when you are fasting. Second, you are going to burn food when you are eating. The fact is that you do not have to worry about starving as this takes much longer than the maximum 20 hours that you will go without food. Intermittent fasting tricks the body into thinking its starving, allowing you to experience many of the benefits to the metabolism being in this state has for the body, without any of the downsides.

With intermittent fasting, the longest you would go without eating is about 20 hours rather than 3 days, and most of the fasting occurs while you are sleeping. As such, it's practically impossible for intermittent fasting to damage your metabolism in the long-term.

Don't I need to eat every few hours to avoid hunger or blood sugar issues?

This is a common misconception. We have been led to believe that if we do not eat every 2-3 hours, we are going to get overly hungry or we will experience hypoglycemia from not eating. Unless you have an issue with diabetes that needs to be treated by a doctor, there is no reason that skipping a meal or two, or even fasting will result in this.

The reason that you feel hungry every few hours is that you have trained your body to be hungry frequently. The steady stream of carbs makes life easy on the body because it never has to go through and use its reserves to keep you energized. However, this often results in you gaining weight and holding onto the fat around your body. Fasting has a suppressive effect on your hunger and you will be able to eat larger portions when you break your fast which helps to satisfy your appetite. You may run into some issues of hunger during the first few days, but once you get past that, you will be fine.

What if I get hungry?

You will probably feel hungry when you first get started with intermittent fasting. This is because the body is used to having a steady stream of carbs to use for fuel and you have suddenly forced it to change its pattern. Your job during the fast, however, it to make it through until you are allowed to eat again. After a few days, you will be able to go on these fasts without feeling as hungry, and it won't take long until you are able to see the results.

Now, if you are on one of these fasts and you find that you are really hungry and want to break that fast, there are a few things that you should keep in mind:

- *Drink more water*: Sometimes, it's not hunger that is going to ruin your plans but thirst. Consider drinking a few glasses of water and see how you feel.

- *Simmer down*: It's only a short period of time until you can eat again. Think of how accomplished you will feel when you are done and how much better you will feel as a result.

- *Stay busy*: Sometimes, you are just hungry because you are sitting around and not doing anything. If you are having cravings or feel hungry, it's time to get up and move. Go to work, read a book, go for a walk, or do something that will keep you busy.

- *Discipline*: Fasting is no harder to do than some of the other diet plans that you may try. Try to stay consistent for at least a month before you make any other decisions as a result.

Are there any disadvantages to intermittent fasting?

There are many great benefits to fasting! You will be able to get your blood sugars in line, feel more energized, and have more time because you are not meal planning all the time. However, there are also a few side effects that you will need to pay attention to. For example, some people complain that they deal with nausea and headaches when they first get started with an intermittent fast. These will usually go away after a few days and can be helped by drinking more water. You may also need to go to the bathroom more often because most people increase their fluid intake when they are on a fast.

Can I stay on intermittent fasting long term?

Yes, this is a plan that you can stay on long term. And, once you get the hang of how fasting works, you are going to naturally want to stick with it because it's so easy. Intermittent fasting is not so much a diet as it is a plan for when you are able to eat and when you shouldn't. It will help you to burn fat and lose weight with less work.

Which fast should I go with?

You can choose the fast that works best for you and your lifestyle; each of can be efficient and will help you lose weight in no time. What it ultimately boils down to is personal preference and what works best for your schedule. Ideally, you will be able to find a type of intermittent fasting that works with your existing schedule because having to adapt your life around the idea of fasting just means adding another layer of difficultly to forming a new habit in the first place.

What happens if I have trouble staying on this fast?

Beginning a new lifestyle change can take some time, but the number one thing that you can do is make sure that you stick with it. Trying the intermittent fast for one day and assuming it doesn't work because you do not see immediate results is one of the worst things that you can do. Keep in mind that it takes a full 30 days to build a new habit, which means you need to stick with it for at least a month before you can hope to see your results with any degree of accuracy.

With that said, if you are having a hard time getting the intermittent fasting habit to stick, finding someone who can hold you accountable is a great way to get started and stat consistent. See if you are able to find an online community of people who would like to work with you to hold you accountable, if not, even having a friend that you report to might be enough to get the habit to stick. While you certainly don't need other people around to ensure you lose weight, they can make it much easier to stay on course.

Conclusion

Thanks for making it through to the end of this book. Hopefully, you found it an enjoyable way to learn about intermittent fasting and meeting your weight loss goals once and for all.

The next step is to take some time to get on an intermittent fast. There is so much that you can learn about this fasting method, and it's a great way for you to easily lose weight while still eating most of the things you love in moderation. Whether you have tried weight loss plans in the past or are just getting started, this guidebook will help you get started with intermittent fasting. If the information provided in the previous chapters work for you, there is no reason you shouldn't be able to find the results you are looking for thanks to intermittent fasting.

Review Request

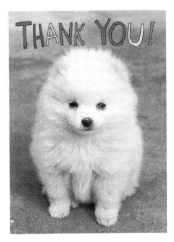

If you enjoyed this book or found it useful, then I'd like to ask you for a quick favor: would you be kind enough to leave a review for this book on Amazon? It'd be greatly appreciated.

Your feedback does matter and helps me to make improvements so I can provide the best content possible. Thank you!

You can leave a review here:

Thank you for your support!

Made in the USA
Columbia, SC
29 August 2018